Competency Exam Prep and Review for Nursing Assistants

Competency Exam Prep and Review for Nursing Assistants

Brief Table of Contents

Competency Exam Prep and Review for Nursing Assistants

Contents

> • Indicates a Performance Procedure

Chapter 8:

Chapter 9:

Chapter 10:

Chapter 11:

Chapter 12:

Performance Procedures

Preface

This training manual was developed to comply with the guidelines set by the Department of Health and Human Services in compliance with Public Law 100-203, referred to as the Omnibus Reconciliation Act of 1987 (OBRA). This law requires that nursing assistants (nurse aides) have, at a minimum, 75 hours of training and a complete competency evaluation program.

This manual was designed to serve as a guide to the competency evaluation program. Included in this course is the content required to successfully complete the written and the manual skills components of the examination.

CPR, cardiopulmonary resuscitation, is not included in this curriculum. It is strongly recommended by the author that the CPR and Clearing Obstructed Airway components be taught by a Certified CPR instructor.

Chapters 1 through 7 serve as the initial training. By OBRA standards, this initial training must consist of at least 16 hours. The author feels 16 hours provide only an overview of the content of chapters 1 through 7. Reinforcement of the content in these chapters can be given in succeeding lessons.

This manual is a very basic "need-to-know" text. It is assumed the instructor will draw upon professional experiences with care of the elderly to provide the "nice-to-know" content. Throughout the entire content of this manual, the intent of the OBRA law is supported—to assure residents in the long-term care facility be treated with care, dignity and respect, while assisting residents to attain and maintain the highest possible level of independence.

This exam review manual can be used with additional resources to create a complete training package.

BASIC NURSING PROCEDURES FOR LONG-TERM CARE is a series of 12 video cassettes containing 41 essential clinical skills. The instructor can start clinical training immediately using these high-quality video demonstrations. The procedural steps coordinate with all Delmar competency-based texts for Nursing Assistants.

ESSENTIALS FOR THE NURSING ASSISTANT IN LONG-TERM CARE is a complete text for any 75-90 hour curriculum. This text starts off with 16 hours of initial training and then covers basic and intermediate procedures. It is designed to enhance learning for "average" and "special needs" learners and for those who speak English as a second language. "Essentials" is competency-based with skills checklists to make the required record keeping easier. An Instructional Resource kit is available, providing program management support, learning resources, advanced procedures and advanced content for extended programs; also, materials for working with the disadvantaged learner.

EXAM PREP AND REVIEW FOR NURSING ASSISTANTS The video series can also be used with *Hegner's Assisting in Long-Term Care*, a comprehensive text developed for 100-150 hour programs.

For multi-competency programs, the instructor may choose Cald-well's **NURSING ASSISTANT: A NURSING PROCESS APPROACH** 5E. A comprehensive 4-color text covering both Acute and Long-Term Care Assisting.

COMPETENCY EXAM PREP AND REVIEW has been designed to provide exposure to test-taking using multiple choice questions on a simulation of the Psychological Corp exam layout. A chapter on test-taking techniques will also help the learner build confidence to take the exam and succeed.

For those setting up new programs or applying for state approval, Delmar's **PROGRAM MANAGEMENT FOR NURSING ASSIST-ING** by Doris Nuttelman will provide a thorough guide to ensuring State approval, writing program proposals, preparing a curriculum, and teaching adult and disadvantaged learners. Every page of this manual is practical, including ready-made correlations of state required content to specific page numbers, video locations, for every Delmar nursing assisting publication along with estimated course hours. This is an invaluable tool for starting a quality program in the shortest possible time.

COMPETENCY EXAM PREP AND REVIEW FOR NURSING ASSISTANTS is part of the most comprehensive and flexible training system available. It is hoped these extensive resources will contribute to quality assurance and to job satisfaction and self-esteem for long-term care paraprofessionals. The author and publisher hope their efforts may also improve quality of life for long-term care residents.

About the Author

Barbara Kast is instructor of nursing assistants and health occupa-tions, Northeast Metro Technical College, White Bear Lake, Minneso-ta. Barbara has been Project Consultant for the State of Minnesota Department of Vocational Technical Education in the design and implementation of nursing assistants' curriculum. Barbara is also studying for a master's degree in curriculum at the University of Wis-consin.

Contributors

Eloise Sampson, RN, BSN, MPH, is also an instructor at Northeast Metro Technical College. Ms. Sampson wrote and contributed each review quiz at the end of every chapter as well as the Practice Exam in this book and the Review Exam in the accompanying Instructor's Guide.

Larry J. Bailey, professor, Vocational Education Studies, Southern Illinois University, Carbondale, Illinois, is the author of Appendix A, Test-Taking Methods and Guidelines.

Chapter 1

The Role and Responsibility of the Nursing Assistant

In this chapter you will learn what your role and responsibilities are as a member of the health care team. After reading this chapter you should be able to:

- Define Key Terms
- Describe the Role of the Nursing Assistant
- Describe the Responsibilities of a Nursing Assistant
- Identify Members of the Health Care Team
- Describe Ethics for the Nursing Assistant
- Describe the Resident's Care Plan
- Describe Individualized Care
- Identify the Changes that Occur in Normal Aging

Key Terms

Care plan: A written plan of care for an individual resident

Charge nurse: The person responsible for the resident's care during a certain work period

Continuity of care: The process by which the care of a resident continues uninterrupted, using the same methods toward that resident's goals

Dignity: The state of being respected or held in honor or esteem

Ethics: A moral code that guides a person's behavior

Etiquette: Being polite, courteous, and kind towards others

Geriatrics: Related to the aged or the aging process and diseases of the elderly

Job description: A list of duties and responsibilities involved in a particular job

Long-term care facility: A nursing home or place where people provide services to others

L.P.N. or L.V.N.: Licensed Practical Nurse or Licensed Vocational Nurse. One who has completed one year of nursing school and passed a state licensing examination for practical nurses

Nursing assistant, Nurse aide: A person who provides nursing or nursing related services to persons in health care facilities who is supervised by a nurse

Resident: A person living in his or her own home, a nursing home, or other long-term care facility

Registered nurse: A person who has completed 2 to 4 years of nursing school and passed a state examination for registered nurses

The Role of Nursing Assistants

Welcome to the health care field! You are about to become a member of a growing industry where your work can give you great personal satisfaction. As a **nursing assistant**, sometimes called a nurse aide, you can help others while achieving your own personal growth. The nursing assistant is a person working in a health care setting to help the nurse give personal care to a resident, patient, or client (Figure 1-1).

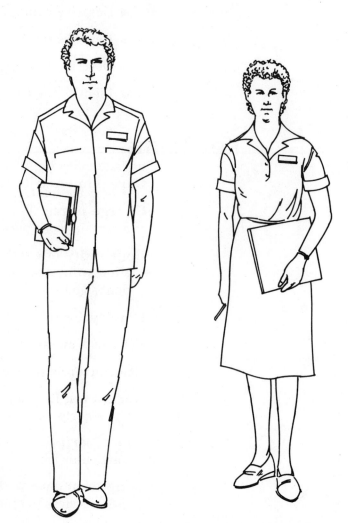

FIGURE 1-1.
Either men or women may have a satisfying career as a nursing assistant.

Health Care Facilities

Health care facilities can be separated into two groups: those that give acute care and those that give less acute care, usually for a long time. Hospitals are an example of acute care facilities, where persons usually stay for a short period of time. Long-term care facilities usually have persons staying for a long period of time, sometimes for years. **Long-term care facilities** are referred to by different names such as convalescent home, nursing home or residence, care center, care facility, or other names. The people who reside in these long-term care facilities are called **residents**. Many of the residents in a nursing home are elderly, although there may be younger residents requiring personal care. Since the term **geriatrics** means care of the elderly, you may be referred to as a geriatric aide. This book is designed to prepare you to work in a long-term care facility.

Nurse as Supervisor

As a nursing assistant you will be supervised by a nurse. The nurse may be either a **Registered Nurse (R.N.)** or a **Licensed Practical Nurse (L.P.N.)** or **Licensed Vocational Nurse (L.V.N.).** Your assignment of work duties and what residents you are to provide care for will be made by your supervising nurse, sometimes called the head nurse or **charge nurse**. This nurse is to whom you will ask questions and report anything about the resident. You are a part of the nursing service department in the long-term care facility.

Personal Qualifications

Since your role as a nursing assistant is giving personal care to others, you must have certain qualities and personal characteristics. Some important qualifications for a nursing assistant to be successful are the following:

- A sincere interest in working with people

- An attitude of respect towards the elderly

- A belief in the dignity of each person

- An ability to control one's emotions

- Honesty, reliability, and dependability

- Willingness to accept direction

- A patient, cheerful, and sensitive nature

- A clean and neat appearance

- Good health—A nursing assistant must stand and walk a lot as well as lift and move people

The Responsibilities of Nursing Assistants _____

The responsibilities of the nursing assistant are usually spelled out in detail in a job description. A **job description** will be given to you by your employer or boss. The description details the particular tasks you are expected to do in that facility. This may vary from one health care facility to another. Remember, everything you do is under the supervision of the nurse.

Job Description

Your job description will list the duties and tasks you are expected to do and may include such things as the following:

- Helping the resident with personal care, such as bathing, mouth care, grooming, dressing, toileting, and skin care

- Helping the resident to eat and drink

- Caring for the resident's environment

- Maintaining safety for the resident

- Taking and recording vital signs

- Observing and reporting abnormal signs and symptoms

- Caring for the resident who is dying

- Measuring height and weight

- Measuring food and fluid intake

- Lifting, moving, turning, and transferring residents

- Helping the resident with equipment or devices such as hearing aids

- Helping the resident to maintain the rights guaranteed by the "Resident's Bill of Rights"

- Helping the resident with mental health needs

- Performing record keeping as indicated by the facility

- Doing other tasks as assigned

The policies of facilities vary, but generally you are expected to care for any resident in the facility. Male and female nursing assistants are usually expected to care for residents of both sexes. If this concerns you, talk to the employer before accepting the job.

Long-term care facilities usually require nursing assistants to wear a uniform. The type of uniform you must wear will be decided by your employer. The uniform often includes a name tag that must be worn. It is your responsibility to follow the facility's policy regarding the uniform code.

Dependability is an important quality of any employee but especially so in health care. For this reason it is important that you remain healthy, so you can be depended upon to be at work. It is your responsibility to let your employer know when you are ill and cannot report to work.

Job Limitations

The nursing assistant has certain job limitations. There are some tasks the nursing assistant does not do. These too will vary from one health care facility to another but generally the following tasks are job limitations. Nursing assistants:

- Do not give medications

- Do not take orders from the doctor

- Do not perform any procedures they have not been taught

- Do not perform any tasks forbidden by the policy of the institution

Whenever you are not sure of a task or procedure, always ask the supervising nurse for help.

The Health Care Team

As a nursing assistant, you are part of a very important team. The goal of the entire staff of long-term care facilities is to provide the best care possible for the resident. This requires cooperation of all staff members (Figure 1-2).

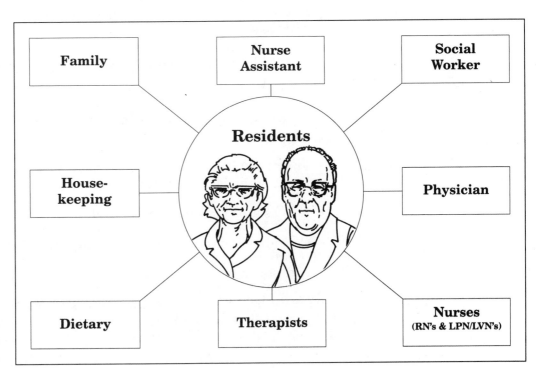

FIGURE 1-2. The health care team.

The team contributing to the resident's care includes the following:

- the resident

- the physician

- the nursing staff

- staff members from the various therapy departments, including physical, occupational, speech, and activity therapy

- social workers

- dietary staff

- housekeeping and maintenance staff members

- office and administrative staff persons

- and others

Ethics for the Nursing Assistant

Ethics is part of a moral code that guides the behavior of the health care worker. Ethics is making judgments about what is right and what is wrong. An ethical nursing assistant is one who:

- Promotes health, independence, safety, and quality of life for each resident

- Respects each resident as an individual

- Understands and follows all the principles covered by the "Resident's Bill of Rights"

- Respects the resident's area as the private space of that resident, and treats the personal belongings of the resident with care

- Keeps information confidential

- Respects the resident's right to privacy

- Has a positive attitude toward the facility in which one is employed

- Functions as a member of the health care team working within limits of the job description

- Acts as a responsible employee at all times

- Considers the resident's needs to be most important

- Accepts no money, or "tips or favors", for service to the resident

- Has a polite, courteous, and kind attitude to residents, visitors, and other staff members

Resident's Care Plan

Upon admission to a long-term care facility a **care plan** for each resident is developed. This plan must be in written form. It is developed in a staff conference where the resident and the resident's family are invited (Figure 1-3). The long- and short-term goals are defined as well as who is responsible for carrying out these goals. A care plan assures that the resident will have continuity of care. This plan must be updated and reviewed regularly. As a nursing assistant, you are responsible for knowing what your job is and how it relates to the care plan. It is your job to ask your supervisor about anything you do not understand.

An important responsibility you have as a nursing assistant is to notice any changes in the resident. Any changes must be reported to the supervising nurse. When observing and reporting, you must be accurate. It is better to report too much than to forget to report something.

Individualized Care

The nursing home is home to many different types of residents. Because patients stay in hospitals for a shorter amount of time, we are seeing residents come to the long-term care facility to complete their recovery. Many long-term care facilities are developing special units for these residents. You may find one facility that specializes in rehabilitation, another that provides care for residents with mental

NURSING CARE PLAN SUMMARY

Person To Be Contacted If Emergency:
TURNER, AUDRY — 762-5005
Name — Phone
684 PARK ST. DALLAS, TEXAS
Address

Name — Phone

Address

Pastor, Rabbi, Priest:
REV. BRUCE WILLIAMS — 762-5872
Name — Phone
419 BRIGHT ST. (PROT.)
Address

Social Security No. 024-14-4282
Medicaid No. M-682-6881
Medicare No. 024-14-4282

Former Occupation, Hobbies or Interests:
OFFICE MANAGER - READING, KNITTING, BOWLING

Funeral Home/Donor Institution:

Name — Phone

Address

BH 24
Rev. 10-81

NAME WALLACE, ELEANOR — Room 16B — Date 9/8/

INTAKE
		Chair	Bed	Out of Room
___ Feeds Self	B	✓		✓
✓ Feed - Help	D			
___ Feed Patient	S			
___ Nourishment				

OUTPUT
Urinary
✓ Continent ___ Incont. ___ Catheter
Bowel
✓ Continent ___ Incont. ___ Colostomy

ACTIVITY
ASST. Up - Ad Lib ___ Chair ___ Stretcher
___ Stand ___ Lift ___ Am't Help
___ Walk - Self ✓ Walk - Help MOD. Am't Help
Passive Exercises LEFT ARM LEFT LEG
Restraint (Type)
___ Always ___ As Needed In Bed
___ Always ___ As Needed In Chair

HYGIENE
Century Tub Bath M - F days/time
Bed Bath ___ days/time
Teeth ___ Natural ✓ Artificial
Shampoo - Beauty Shop THURS. 10 AM days/time
- Century Tub ___ Regular Shampoo ___ Special Shampoo

THERAPY
Physical Therapy WED. - SAT. 9:30 A.M. days/time
Speech Therapy MONDAY 3:00 P.M. days/time
Activities - Group TUES. - THURS. 1:00 P.M. days/time
- Individual ___ days/time

OTHER
___ Hearing Problem
___ Sight Problem
✓ Speech Problem
___ Behavior Problem
___ Other

SHORT TERM GOAL - IMPROVE MOBILITY AND SPEECH SKILLS.
LONG TERM GOAL - DISCHARGE TO HOME CARE.

FIGURE 1-3. Example of a resident's Care Plan.

health problems such as Alzheimer's disease or that may care for AIDS patients. Some long-term care facilities do not specialize and admit persons with any type of disability. The reasons for admission to the long-term care facility may vary widely, which emphasizes the importance of individualized care for each resident.

Although the residents' ages vary a lot, often the majority of the residents are elderly. For many reasons people live longer today than ever before in our nation. As one ages, the resistance to disease, stress, and injury decreases. Therefore the elderly are more likely to need help in meeting their personal needs. It is very important that each resident be treated as an individual. Remember the following in giving individualized care to residents:

- Each resident is a separate person with different needs and wants

- Assist residents to become and remain independent

- Maintain resident's dignity by treating the resident as an adult at all times. Allowing residents to do as much as possible adds to dignity and self worth

- Offer choices whenever possible. This helps the resident maintain a sense of control and adds to his self-esteem

- Be involved with the resident's family and be aware of activity programs that can include family members

- Schedule care to allow resident's participation in activity programs

- Assisting residents to meet their physical, psychosocial and spiritual needs

Normal Aging Process

Since many of the residents in a long-term care facility are elderly, a general understanding of the normal aging process is important for the nursing assistant to know.

Body Systems and Normal Aging

All parts of the body are affected by the normal aging process. When studying the body, we look at it as a group of systems that work together. A body system is a group of organs working together to perform a particular function. A brief overview of body systems and how the aging process affects them follows.

Integumentary System includes the skin, hair, and nails. Sweat and oil glands are part of the exocrine glands.

- Changes in normal aging
  - Skin becomes fragile, tears easily, loses fatty tissue under skin
  - Hair thins and grays
  - Nails thicken and harden
  - Less natural oil and sweat are produced

- Results of normal aging
  - Skin is less resistant to injury
  - Skin bruises more readily
  - Skin becomes drier
  - Tissues heal slower
  - Changes in skin and other systems make body regulation of temperature more difficult. The elderly often complain of feeling cold

Musculoskeletal System includes the bones, muscles and joints.

- Changes in normal aging
  - Bones become porous and brittle
  - Muscles lose strength and bulk
  - Joints and ligaments become less flexible

- Results of normal aging
  - Fractures occur easier
  - Exercise and good nutrition become essential

Digestive System includes the stomach, intestines, and other organs that help digest food.

- Changes in normal aging
  - Digestive system gradually slows down
  - Appetite decreases
  - Constipation often occurs
  - Chewing ability is often decreased

- Results of normal aging
  - Pleasant mealtime environment is required
  - Meals must be attractive and stimulating

Cardiovascular System includes the heart and blood vessels. **Circulatory System** is restricted to the blood vessels.

- Changes in normal aging
  - Cardiac output is reduced
  - Blood vessels become less elastic
  - Heart disease is common in the elderly

- Results of normal aging
  - Person may need to rest more frequently
  - Exercise is necessary to stimulate circulation
  - Blood pressure may be elevated

Respiratory System includes the lungs and air passages.

- Changes in normal aging
  - Exchange of oxygen and carbon dioxide are decreased
  - Lungs lose some elasticity
  - Deep breathing is more difficult for the aged person

- Results of normal aging
  - Respiratory infections are more likely
  - Respiratory changes may make an elderly person more tired
  - Deep breathing should be encouraged

Genitourinary System includes the kidneys and bladder. Another word commonly used is Excretion.

- Changes in normal aging
  - Kidney function is reduced
  - Bladder elasticity decreases
  - Men often have prostate enlargement

- Results of normal aging
  - Bladder emptying is less efficient
  - More urinary infections occur
  - Need to empty bladder is often urgent
  - Coughing and sneezing may cause women to be unable to control urine passage
  - Men may have trouble urinating

Central Nervous System includes the brain and spinal cord. The **Nervous System** involves nerve endings.

- Changes in normal aging
  - Reaction time to stimuli is slower
  - Blood flow to brain is decreased
  - Diseases of these systems may cause physical or mental disability

- Results of normal aging
  - More time is needed when caring for many elderly residents
  - Resident needs more time to make choices

The eyes, ears, nose and taste buds of the mouth are part of the **senses**.

- Changes in normal aging
  - All senses gradually slow down

- Results of normal aging
  - Vision, hearing, and agility are reduced
  - Irritations on skin and feet may go unnoticed due to less sensation or feeling

It is important to become more aware of these normal changes in the aging process. The changes that occur in these body systems will affect the manner of the care needed for each resident.

Generalizations Relating to Normal Aging

You have already learned that each resident is an individual person who must be treated in an individual manner. However, some general statements are true about normal aging:

- All body systems are affected

- Resistance to injury and disease is decreased

- People age at different rates

- All body systems gradually slow down

- The aging process is affected by lifestyle, nutrition, mental, physical, and emotional health, and attitude

Key Points in This Chapter

The nursing assistant provides personal care while working under a nurse's supervision.

The person living in a long-term care facility is the resident.

As a nursing assistant, you are part of the nursing service team.

Good health, honesty, dependability, and sincere desire to work with people are required qualities of a nursing assistant.

The job description is a list of tasks and duties you are expected to perform as a nursing assistant.

Your assignment is made by the nurse and may include working with any resident, male or female.

Cooperation with all members of the health care team is an important part of your role.

The care plan is a written plan describing long- and short-term goals for resident care.

Each resident is an individual and must be treated with respect and dignity.

The normal aging process occurs in all people at different rates.

All body systems gradually slow down.

The Role and Responsibility of the Nursing Assistant

Choose the best answer for the questions below.

1. Nursing assistants are sometimes called

   (A) nurse aides.
   (B) nurse helpers.
   (C) practical nurses.
   (D) registered nurses.

2. Which of the following is true about long-term care facilities?

   (A) Persons stay in these facilities a short time.
   (B) Persons stay in these facilities while recovering from surgery.
   (C) Persons stay in these facilities for a long time.
   (D) Persons are admitted to these facilities with acute illnesses.

3. Persons living in long-term care facilities are called

   (A) senior citizens.
   (B) patients.
   (C) retired.
   (D) residents.

4. Which term means care of the elderly?

   (A) Resident
   (B) Geriatrics
   (C) Medical
   (D) Nursing

5. Who is the supervisor of the nursing assistant?

   (A) Doctor
   (B) Administrator
   (C) Nurse
   (D) Family

6. Which department in the long-term care facility is the nursing assistant a part of?

   (A) Administration
   (B) Nursing
   (C) Maintenance
   (D) Dietary

7. Which of the following qualifications are necessary for the nursing assistant?

   (A) Honesty
   (B) Reliability
   (C) Dependability
   (D) All of the above

8. The responsibilities of a nursing assistant are detailed in a

   (A) job description.
   (B) job manual.
   (C) job list.
   (D) résumé.

9. Some of the tasks and duties you will be expected to perform include

   (A) assisting residents in personal care.
   (B) feeding residents.
   (C) giving medications.
   (D) All of the above
   (E) A and B only

10. Male and female nursing assistants will

   (A) be expected to care for residents of either sex.
   (B) care for only same sex residents.
   (C) work only with nursing assistants of the same sex.
   (D) work on separate sections of the facility.

11. Part of the uniform you will wear will include

   (A) a name tag.
   (B) anti-static shoes.
   (C) caps or hats.
   (D) isolation gowns.

12. Which of the following is *not* a responsibility of the nursing assistant?

   (A) Bathing and dressing residents
   (B) Taking telephone orders from the doctor
   (C) Taking and recording temperatures
   (D) Caring for the dying resident

13. What should you do if you are not certain of a task you are told to do?

   (A) Ask another nursing assistant to do it for you
   (B) Tell your nurse you are uncertain and ask for help
   (C) Forget about doing the task
   (D) Do the task anyway

14. Which of the following is *not* included in the health care team of the long-term facility?

   (A) The nursing staff
   (B) Social workers
   (C) Dietary staff
   (D) Hospital staff

15. A written plan listing long- and short-term goals for the resident and who is responsible for assisting in these goals is the

   (A) job description.
   (B) assignment sheet.
   (C) team report.
   (D) care plan.

16. Which of the following statements is true regarding the normal aging process?

   (A) All persons become unable to heal properly after injury at age 65.
   (B) Only the skin of the elderly is affected by aging.
   (C) All body systems gradually slow down.
   (D) All persons show signs of aging the same way.

17. The normal aging process will cause nails to become

   (A) thin and weak.
   (B) thick and hard.
   (C) loose from the nailbed.
   (D) discolored and yellow.

18. Ethical behavior on the part of the nursing assistant means to

   (A) know what is right and what is wrong.
   (B) practice good body mechanics.
   (C) work with other health team members.
   (D) work on the weekends.

ANSWERS
1. A
2. C
3. D
4. B
5. C
6. B
7. D
8. A
9. E
10. A
11. A
12. B
13. B
14. D
15. D
16. C
17. B
18. A

Chapter 2
Basic Human Needs

In this chapter you will learn the importance of basic human needs and ways you can help residents meet these needs. After reading this chapter you should be able to:

- Define Key Terms

- Describe Basic Human Needs/Physical and Psychological

- Identify Developmental Tasks Associated with the Aging Process

- Identify Coping Mechanisms for Grief and Loss

- Describe Death and Dying

- Demonstrate Postmortem Care

Key Terms

Coping mechanisms: The methods people use or develop to cope with or handle stress

Physiological needs: Physical human needs

Postmortem care: Care given the body after death

Psychological needs: The emotional, spiritual, and mental needs of humans

Self-actualization: The state of having achieved one's full potential or ability

Self-esteem: Satisfaction with oneself

Spiritual needs: The needs having to do with one's spiritual or religious beliefs

Therapeutic: Serving to cure, heal, or preserve health

Human Needs

All people have the same basic human needs, regardless of age, sex, position, or status in life. Some needs, however, come first before other needs. For example, breathing is more important than eating, even though both are necessary to live. When our body's basic needs are met, we move up to higher levels of needs, such as safety and security and love and belonging (Figure 2-1). These basic needs are what motivate people to behave as they do (Figure 2-2).

Knowledge of the basic needs will help you understand and give better care to the resident. It may be that the resident who is always calling for attention is not having met the need for love and belonging. Many residents in the long-term care facility will need help in meeting basic human needs.

Basic human needs can be grouped into two categories: physical and psychological. Physical needs are called **Physiological**. These are needs having to do with the body and are necessary for survival.

Other needs involve the emotional, spiritual or mental relationships of humans. The terms to describe this emotional type of need are **Psychological** or **Psychosocial**.

All the basic human needs are equally important. These needs must be somewhat met for a person to be a healthy person. Learning about ways to meet these needs will help you give quality care to each resident.

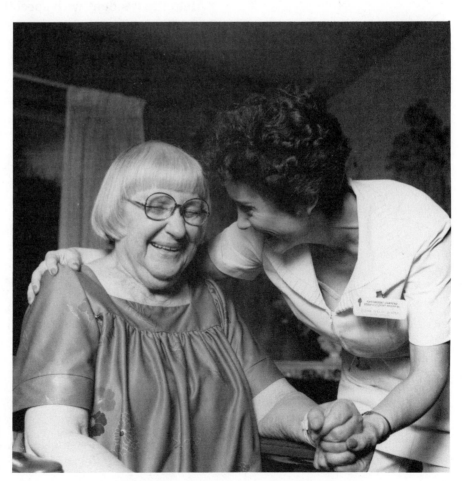

FIGURE 2-1.
Nursing assistants and residents can find joy in their time together.

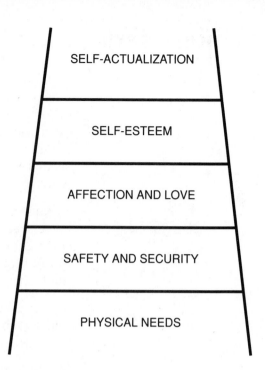

FIGURE 2-2.
Hierarchy or "ladder" of basic human needs.

Physical Needs and Ways to Help the Resident Meet These Needs

- ○ Food
  - Make mealtime as pleasant as possible
  - Help the resident to eat
  - Help the resident with special foods
  - Feed the resident when necessary
  - Assist the nurse with feeding tubes or intravenous infusions when necessary

- ○ Oxygen, air
  - Elevate head of bed for resident with breathing problems
  - Properly position bed and chairs
  - Assist residents to ambulate, or walk, or exercise frequently as indicated on care plan
  - Make sure clothing or other garments do not fit to tightly
  - Assist with oxygen therapy when necessary

- ○ Water
  - Offer fluids frequently, especially in hot weather
  - Keep water containers within reach

- ○ Elimination, toileting
  - Assist resident in toileting needs
  - Provide privacy during elimination
  - Being calm or unemotional in response to resident who is unable to control urine or stool passage

- ○ Rest
  - Assist in bedtime or sleep preparation
  - Recognize any changes in sleep patterns

- ○ Activity and exercise
  - Encourage range-of-motion exercise in ADLs
  - Ambulate, transfer, and move residents properly

- Assist resident to participate in activities of choice
- Encourage resident to be as independent as possible when it is consistent with care plan

○ Stimulation
  - Encourage involvement in activities available at facility
  - Take time to listen to resident and encourage talking by resident
  - Place resident in area where there is activity to observe
  - Do not isolate resident

○ Sexuality
  - Encourage use of appropriate clothing, cosmetics, and hair styles to maintain sexual identity (Figure 2-3)
  - Compliment the resident on his or her attractiveness
  - Provide privacy to couples expressing intimacy needs. Knock before entering rooms
  - Respond nicely to a resident who is masturbating. Take the resident to his or her room. Respond in nonjudgmental manner, and do not shame or make resident feel guilty or foolish

Safety and Security Needs and Ways to Help the Resident Meet These Needs

○ Safety
  - Keep area safe and free of hazards
  - Use physical restraints when ordered
  - Follow the care plan for release and exercise of resident who has physical restraints

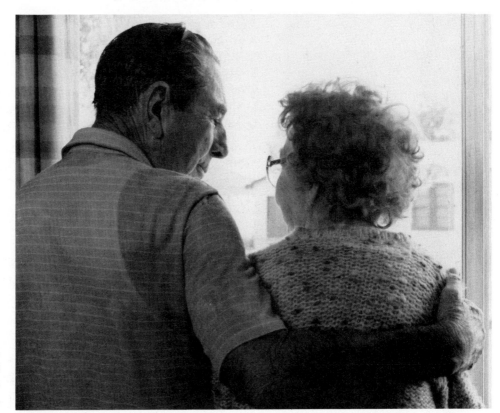

FIGURE 2-3.
The need to express one's sexuality is present in people of all ages.

- Keep call light within reach of resident
- Know the tasks you perform
- Be alert to safety at all times
- Use lifting aids and transfer belts when indicated

○ Security
- Respect the resident's belongings
- Help resident adjust to new surroundings, other residents, and staff persons
- Reassure resident, providing physical and mental support
- Welcome family and friends
- Provide privacy. Knock on doors and wait for response before entering
- Maintain confidentiality when the resident tells you something

Love and Belonging Needs and Ways to Help the Resident Meet These Needs

○ Caring about someone
- Listen to resident, but do not hurry him or her. Encourage talk of past when appropriate
- Show interest in resident's family and past experiences
- Encourage contact with other residents
- Ask nurse or social worker for information about the resident's past life, if this information will assist in resident's care
- Realize some residents may have close friends who are not family members

○ Being cared about
- Show interest in resident
- Touch resident in kind and gentle manner
- Show kindness and consideration
- Be kind and friendly to resident's visitors and family
- Inform and encourage family and friends to attend activities
- Family members are often invited to participate in care conference
- Be patient and understanding when interacting with the resident
- Treat the resident as you would wish to be treated
- Allow resident to cry if resident has need to cry. Stay with resident if resident asks

Self-esteem and Ways to Help the Resident Meet This Need

○ Sense of identity and self-esteem
- Always call the resident by the name the resident requests
- Include resident and family in talks about care

- Allow privacy when requested. Knock on doors and wait for response before entering
- Give choices whenever possible. If it is not against care plan, give the resident what is asked for
- If the resident's choice is against the care plan, tell your supervising nurse
- Respect resident's choice in clothing
- Respect individual differences in culture, heredity, interests, and values

○ Feeling important and worthwhile
- Recognize resident's accomplishments, praise freely if appropriate
- Acknowledge resident at all times
- Respect the resident's property and personal items
- Talk to the resident as an adult
- Encourage resident's independence, if consistent with care plan
- Allow resident to do as much as possible; adds to self-esteem
- Encourage the resident's involvement in activity programs. Schedule care to allow resident's participation in activities of choice
- Show interest in family members
- Be courteous to family members. Suggest their continued involvement and visits with resident

Self-Actualization and Ways to Help the Resident Meet This Need

○ **Self-actualization** is the state of having reached one's highest potential or ability in life. It is also a feeling of being satisfied with oneself.
- Look for the resident's strengths, and praise him or her when appropriate
- Support hobbies, interests, and awareness of current events
- Encourage and praise accomplishments
- Take time to appreciate the "history" of the resident

○ Spirituality
- Listen to resident's concerns
- Respect the resident's religious beliefs (Figure 2-4)
- Plan care so that resident can be involved in religious activities of choice
- Provide privacy for religious visiting
- Respect and handle with care religious symbols, pictures, or other objects
- If the resident asks to see any member of the clergy, refer request to nurse

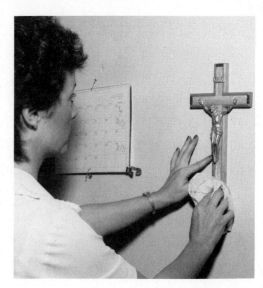

FIGURE 2-4.
The resident has a right to have
religious beliefs.

Developmental Tasks

Theorists suggest that as one matures from infancy to old age, he or she must pass through several stages. During each stage developmental tasks that help you grow must be accomplished in order to mature in a healthy manner. Realize that this theory is general. Not all people mature in these stages in the same way.

An understanding of the normal adult developmental tasks will help you understand the residents you care for. The stages and developmental tasks of the adult are grouped into three categories: early adulthood, middle adulthood, and late adulthood.

- ○ Early adulthood— the late teens to the thirties.
  The developmental tasks in this age group are:
  - Establishing personal and economic independence from parents
  - Developing a career
  - Making a commitment in a relationship
  - Establishing a family

- ○ Middle adulthood— the thirties to the mid-sixties.
  The developmental tasks in this age group are:
  - Expanding personal and social involvement and responsibility
  - Adjusting to the physiological changes of middle age
  - Reaching and maintaining satisfaction in one's career
  - Observing the maturation or growing of children

- ○ Late adulthood—the mid-sixties until death.
  The developmental tasks in this age group are:
  - Adjusting to decreasing physical strengths
  - Adjusting to losses
  - Accepting one's past
  - Realizing and accepting one's mortality

Grief and Loss

When a person experiences a loss, he or she goes through a grief process. You probably have experienced the grief process if you lost a pet or moved to a new school. Imagine how much more difficult it is to lose a loved one. The grief process involves five steps: denial, anger, bargaining, depression and acceptance (Figure 2-5). Because the grief process varies with each of us, not all persons experience each step and not all steps are obvious to others.

The resident in the long-term care facility has had to experience many losses. An understanding of some of the coping mechanisms people use to deal with losses and stress in life will help you understand your residents.

Coping mechanisms are responses to stress that a person uses to protect feelings of self-esteem. Coping mechanisms develop throughout life. The success or failure in gaining positive coping skills depends largely on how well the developmental tasks of earlier life have been done. When the coping ability of a person is strained or inadequate, the following reactions may be seen:

- Chronic complaining

- Agitation

- Restlessness

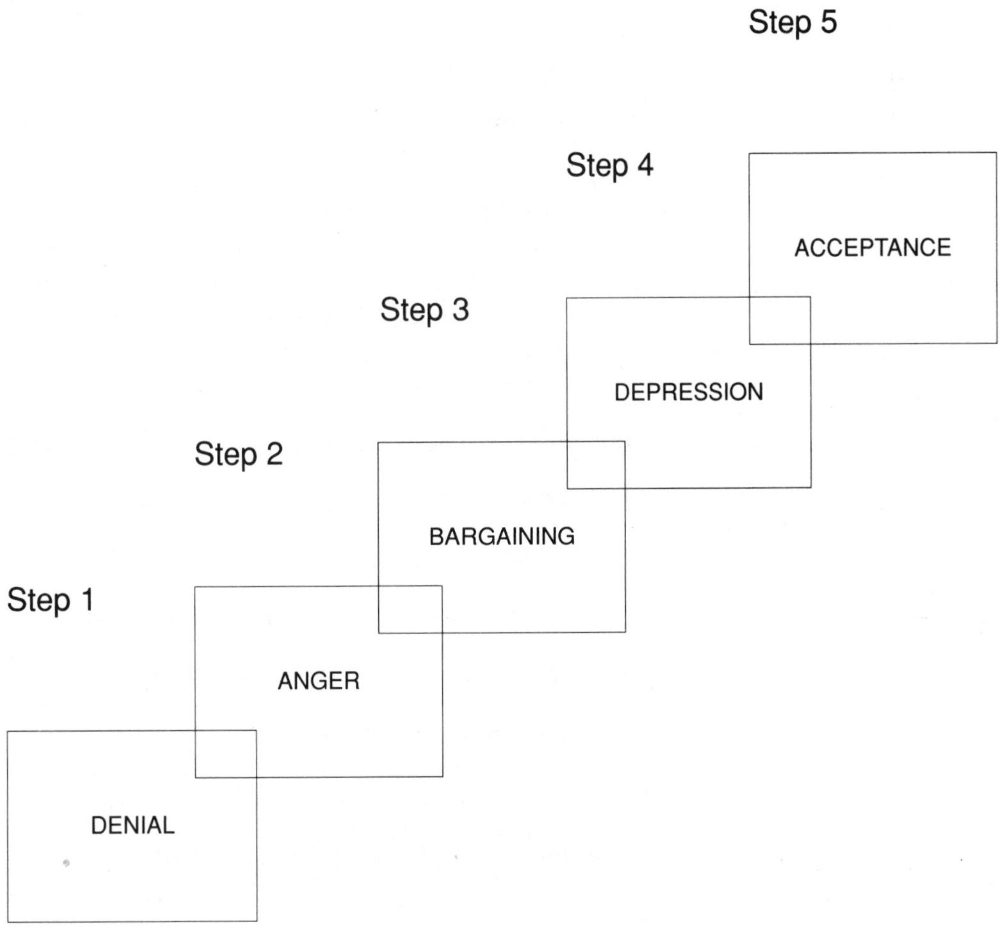

Step 5

Step 4

ACCEPTANCE

Step 3

DEPRESSION

Step 2

BARGAINING

Step 1

ANGER

DENIAL

FIGURE 2-5.
The five steps of
grief or loss.

- Depression

- Withdrawal

- Weight loss or gain

- Sleep disturbances

Residents who react this way often need additional emotional support. Your understanding of basic human needs, normal adult development tasks and coping mechanisms will help you provide quality care for the resident. The following are other ways the nursing assistant can provide this support:

- Use the **therapeutic** communication

- Give the resident choices whenever possible

- Realize angry outbursts from the resident are often the result of feelings of hopelessness or losses experienced

- Direct the resident's emotional energy in positive ways. Encourage activity programs

- Always report any change in resident's behavior to the nurse in charge

Death and Dying

You will be working with persons in the long-term care facility who are near death. Remember, death is a part of living. Death comes to all living things. Many persons look at death as a frightening time. Studies of people who had near-death experiences have shown that death is not unpleasant or frightening. Interviews with many elderly persons showed they have little fear of death. As a nursing assistant in a long-term care facility, dealing with death-related issues may be part of your job. Discussing your own fears of death may help you better understand death and dying. Caring for the person when death is near, as well as caring for the body after death, will probably be included in your responsibility.

Some of the physical signs indicating death is near are the following:

- Pale, moist and cool skin

- A dusky color may appear on lips and fingertips

- Rapid, weak and thready pulse

- Slow, labored, and irregular breathing

- Falling blood pressure

- Involuntary discharge of urine and feces

- Eyes that do not respond to light

The nursing care for the dying resident is continuation of care that shows dignity and respect. Some other points to remember while caring for the dying resident are the following:

- Check care plan for special instructions, or ask the nurse

- Keep the resident clean and comfortable

- Moisten lips and mouth as directed

- Touch and continue to talk to the resident

- Say only things you want the resident to hear. The sense of hearing may be present even if it does not seem so

- Support family members. Allow them to be involved in care, if appropriate

Postmortem Care

If you are to prepare the body after death, refer to your facility's policy on **postmortem** care, or ask the nurse any questions you have. Some facilities have a morgue to which the body is taken. In other facilities the body will be transferred to a mortuary.

Procedure 1
Postmortem Care

1. Wash your hands.

2. Gather supplies: shroud kit with gown and identification tags, basin of warm water, washcloth, towels, and gloves.

3. Give privacy.

4. Treat the body with respect.

5. Wear gloves.

6. Close the eyes by gently pulling eyelids down over eyes.

7. Place cleaned dentures in mouth.

8. Close the mouth. A rolled up washcloth may be placed under chin to keep jaw closed.

9. Remove all tubing from body.

10. Bathe the body, comb hair, and straighten arms and legs.

11. Apply clean dressings to wounds, if necessary.

12. Pad the genital area.

13. Put shroud or gown on body.

14. Attach identification tag to body as indicated by facility policy.

15. Replace any soiled linen.

16. Tidy area of unit.

17. Collect all belongings, place them in bag, and label them correctly. Usually these are given to the resident's family.

18. Give privacy to the family when they visit the body.

19. Follow facility policy, if necessary, to bring body to morgue.

20. Clean unit as directed after body has been removed.

(See Procedure Review, page 203)

Key Points in This Chapter

- All people have the same basic human needs, though some people may express their needs in different ways.

- Physical needs, called physiological needs, refer to the needs of the body.

- Psychological or psychosocial needs refer to the emotional or mental needs of persons.

- Developmental tasks must be somewhat accomplished in order to mature in a healthy manner.

- Coping mechanisms are used and developed in life to cope with stresses.

- The grieving process is a series of five stages that a person experiences after suffering a loss.

- The dying or dead resident must be cared for with the same respect and dignity given all residents.

Review Quiz Chapter 2
Basic Human Needs

Choose the best answer for the questions below.

1. Which of the following statements is true?

   (A) All people have the same basic human needs.
   (B) The basic human needs of people vary according to age.
   (C) Men and women have very different basic human needs.
   (D) All people express their basic needs exactly in the same way.

2. What are psychosocial or psychological needs?

   (A) Needs having to do with the physical body.
   (B) Needs having to do with mental and emotional needs.
   (C) Needs having to do with food, air, and exercise.
   (D) Needs having to do with elimination.

3. Nursing assistants can assist the resident to meet the need for food by

   (A) keeping the head of the bed elevated.
   (B) doing range-of-motion exercises for the resident.
   (C) making mealtime as pleasant as possible.
   (D) providing privacy when doing any personal care.

4. The resident's need for exercise and activity can be met by

   (A) assisting the resident to eat.
   (B) assisting the resident to ambulate.
   (C) taking the resident to the bathroom every 3 hours.
   (D) keeping the resident in bed as much as possible.

5. The nursing assistant can help meet the resident's need for sexuality expression by

   (A) dressing the resident in clothing that is appropriate for his or her sex.
   (B) providing privacy for couples who have intimacy needs.
   (C) telling the resident who is seen masturbating to stop that immediately.
   (D) All of the above
   (E) A and B only

6. The resident's need for love and belonging can be met by

   (A) Keeping the head of the bed up when bathing the resident.
   (B) showing interest and listening closely to the resident.
   (C) making sure equipment is working properly.
   (D) keeping the resident alone most of the time.

7. What is your best response when the resident you are caring for begins to cry?

   (A) Let the resident cry and ask if there is something you can do to help him or her.
   (B) Give the resident a tissue and leave the room.
   (C) Tell the resident, "Stop crying, things will get better."
   (D) Allow the resident to cry and call the family immediately.

8. Calling the resident by the name he or she prefers is one way of meeting the need for

   (A) exercise.
   (B) love.
   (C) identity.
   (D) spiritual growth.

9. How can the nursing assistant help the resident meet his or her spiritual needs?

   (A) By respecting the religious belongings of the resident
   (B) By planning your care for the resident so he/she can attend religious services of choice
   (C) By providing privacy for the resident and visiting clergy and chaplain
   (D) All of the above

10. A developmental task of late adulthood is

   (A) developing a career.
   (B) establishing a family.
   (C) accepting one's mortality.
   (D) making commitments in family life.

11. Responses persons develop in life to handle stress are called

   (A) coping mechanisms.
   (B) grief process.
   (C) memory lapses.
   (D) protests.

12. What is the first step in the grief process?

   (A) Anger
   (B) Denial
   (C) Depression
   (D) Acceptance

13. Which of the following is *not* a true statement?

   (A) All people go through the grief process exactly the same way
   (B) People go through the grief process in individual ways
   (C) Not all people will go through each step of the grief process
   (D) The amount of time of the grief process will vary among people

14. When caring for the resident who is dying, you should

   (A) keep the room as dark as possible.
   (B) keep family and visitors away from the dying person.
   (C) continue caring, touching, and talking to the resident.
   (D) never allow the resident to see family members who are crying.

15. Physical signs of approaching death may include

   (A) pale skin.
   (B) weak and rapid pulse.
   (C) eyes that do not respond to light.
   (D) All of above
   (E) B and C only

Chapter 3

Rights of the Resident

In this chapter you will learn about the importance of the Resident's Rights. After reading this chapter you should be able to:

- Define Key Terms

- List Resident's Rights

- Describe Ways to Accommodate the Resident's Right to Make Choices

- Describe Your Role in Helping the Resident to Resolve Grievances

- List Ways You Can Assist the Resident to Participate in Activities

- Describe Care which Maintains a Resident's Dignity

Key Terms

Abuse: Intentional harm or threatened harm to a person's health or welfare

Adaptive equipment: Equipment or supplies used to make a task easier

Confidentiality: Keeping information or facts private

Dignity: The state of being respected or esteemed

Infringe: To remove, take away or make difficult to attain

Nontherapeutic: Not relating to treatment or therapy

Reprisal: An act performed to gain revenge or to punish another

Restraints: Equipment used to protect, support, or hold a person in a particular position

The Resident's Bill of Rights is a federal law that all members of the health care team must respect (Figure 3-1). The purpose and intent of the law is to make sure that all residents of a long-term care facility are treated with dignity and respect. A copy of these rights is given to each person when admitted to a facility.

Generally, residents have the following rights:

- To be accorded **dignity** in their personal relationship with staff

- To receive quality care regardless of race, color, ethnic origin, age, religion, marital status, sexual preference, or disability

- To receive encouragement and support in making personal choices to accommodate individual needs

- To be respected and protected from harm, both physically and verbally

- To be free of **abuse**

- To have privacy during procedures and when requested

- To have **confidentiality** about their medical condition, medical records, and other information relating to their care

- To be addressed by their preferred name

- To have continuity of care

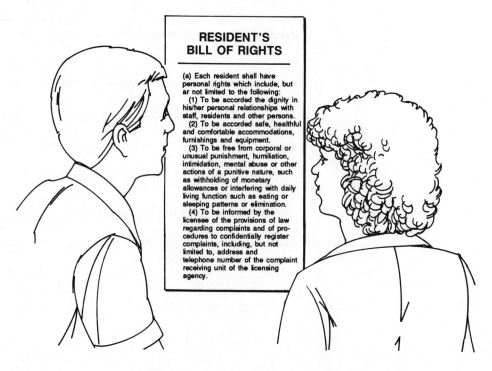

FIGURE 3-1.
Nursing assistants must respect the Resident's Bill of Rights.

- To have personal possessions treated with respect and have them safeguarded

- To have assistance, privacy, and confidentiality in personal communication (mail, telephone calls, visitors, etc.)

- To be informed about the cost and services available

- To refuse treatment. If treatment is refused, an explanation of the likely results of refusal must be given to the resident

- To be free from **nontherapeutic** chemical and physical **restraints**

- To wear their own clothing, keep appropriate personal possessions, and be allowed to spend their own money

- To have family or significant others participate in care conferences

- To receive help in exercising citizenship rights

- To be told the name of the physician responsible for care

- To be informed of the procedures for filing confidential complaints, and for working out complaints. To be given references of available resources

- To participate in religious or political activities if these do not infringe on other resident's rights

These rights give residents the same rights all citizens have. It is part of your role and responsibility to support the resident in exercising these rights. The reason for this law is to promote the interests and well-being of residents in health care facilities. The long-term care facility and its staff must encourage and assist the resident to exercise, or use, these rights.

Some of the ways you, as a nursing assistant, are responsible for seeing the resident's rights are protected are the following:

- Give quality care to all residents, regardless of race, color, ethnic origin, age, religion, handicap, marital status, or sexual preference

- Give privacy when caring for the resident. Knock on doors and wait for answer before entering. Pull privacy curtain when doing care. Cover the sitting resident with a blanket or lap robe, if resident wishes. Give privacy to resident and visitors, if requested

- Keep in confidence all medical information learned about the resident, as well as information learned by phone calls, mail, or visitors. If information learned relates to the condition of the resident, tell the nurse

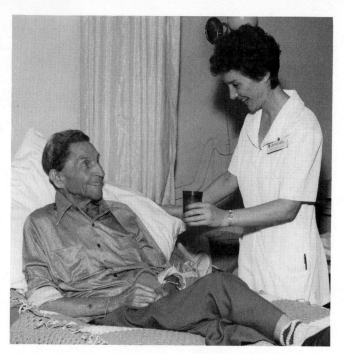

FIGURE 3-2.
Offer choices to the resident whenever possible.

- Call the resident by the name the resident wants to be called

- Help the resident protect any personal possessions

- Help the resident make phone calls or write letters

Resident's Right to Make Choices

One of the statements in the Resident's Bill of Rights gives the resident the right to make personal choices. As a nursing assistant, you often have the most contact with the resident in a long-term care facility. Therefore, you have the most opportunities to assist the resident in making choices (Figure 3-2). Some of the ways you can do this are by:

- Offering choices whenever possible

- Accommodating the resident's requests as to what might be the best time to do certain procedures.

- Taking the time to talk to the resident so you can learn personal preferences

- Talking to the family to learn the resident's interests before his or her admission to the nursing home

- Reporting the resident's preferences to the nurse

A recent study of long-term care facilities showed there are differences in what residents and staff feel is important. This study supports the fact that residents need to be asked what and when they want things done. Remember, this is encouraged by the Resident's Bill of Rights.

Resolving Grievances

A **grievance**, or complaint, occurs when the resident feels his or her rights are **infringed** upon. When this occurs, the resident has a right to file a grievance. The Resident's Bill of Rights gives the resident the right to voice grievances without fear of **reprisal,** or punishment. The policy of your facility will indicate how this procedure is to be carried out. Usually your responsibility is to report the resident's grievance to the nurse, making sure what you report is accurate. Some facilities have a social worker who is responsible for helping resolve grievances (Figure 3-3). Always know and follow the procedure for your facility.

Resident's Participation in Activities

The activity department of a long-term care facility has a very special function. It plans recreational and social functions for the resident. These functions are therapy for the resident. Your role in the activity department is usually that of cooperation. Some of the ways you can help the resident participate in activities are the following:

- Plan your work so the resident can attend the activity of choice

- Be aware of the events planned for the day

- Tell all residents what activities are planned

- Encourage the resident to attend

- Help the resident dress properly, always remembering to allow the resident to do as much self-care as possible.

- Inform the resident's family or friends about activities

- Offer to help the resident get to and from activity programs

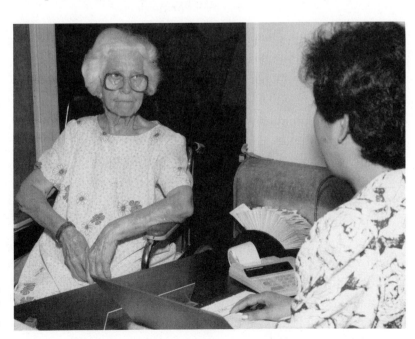

FIGURE 3-3.
The social worker is often responsible for helping the resident file a greivance.

Maintaining Resident's Dignity

There are many ways you can help maintain the resident's dignity. Dignity means having respect for a person. It is important to try to maintain the resident's dignity at all times.

You should realize the resident has had to make many adjustments. Many of these adjustments have been hard and painful. The nursing home resident has suffered many losses and may be angry and frustrated. Remember, the resident once was a younger, active person, so treat the resident as you would want to be treated.

Some of the ways the nursing assistant can help maintain the resident's dignity are the following:

- Maintain an attitude of respect

- Help the resident be as independent as possible. If consistent with the care plan, let the resident do as much as possible for himself

- Use **adaptive** equipment, such as hearing aids, if indicated on the care plan. Teach resident to use the equipment

- Handle personal possessions of the resident with care and security

- Always tell the resident what you are going to do before you do it. Ask permission and cooperation of the resident

- Check with the resident before throwing away any possessions, such as magazines or newspapers

- Refer to the care plan for special instructions, or ask the nurse for information

- Always be alert to safety concerns

- Provide care that protects the resident from abuse, mistreatment, or neglect

- Report any instances of poor care or abuse to the appropriate staff person

Key Points in This Chapter

🔑 The Resident's Bill of Rights is a law that must be respected by all members of the health care facility.

🔑 The Resident's Bill of Rights makes sure the resident is treated with dignity and respect.

🔑 The resident has the right to file a grievance and to be given assistance in doing so.

🔑 The nursing assistant must try to provide privacy for the resident when giving personal care.

🔑 The nursing assistant must cooperate with the activity department in helping the resident do activities of choice.

🔑 Showing respect for the resident includes carefully handling the resident's personal possessions.

🔑 Any abuse or poor care must be reported to the appropriate staff person.

Review Quiz Chapter 3
Rights of the Resident

Choose the best answer for the questions below.

1. A federal law that relates to care of the resident in a long-term care facility is the

   Ⓐ State Guide for Long Term Care Homes.
   Ⓑ Resident's Bill of Rights.
   Ⓒ Ten Amendments.
   Ⓓ Rule and Regulation Guide.

2. The purpose of the Resident's Bill of Rights is to

   Ⓐ limit the cost of health care.
   Ⓑ list the cost of services provided for the resident.
   Ⓒ insure dignity and respect to residents in long-term care facilities.
   Ⓓ provide a document for nursing assistants to charge money for care given.

3. Which of the following is included in the Resident's Bill of Rights?

   Ⓐ To be given privacy when receiving care
   Ⓑ To be told the cost of services
   Ⓒ To receive and send mail
   Ⓓ All of the above

4. When the resident is admitted to the long-term care facility,

   Ⓐ he or she must wear only the clothing issued by the facility.
   Ⓑ he or she should be called by the room number so all staff know there is a new resident.
   Ⓒ a copy of the Resident's Bill of Rights must be given the resident.
   Ⓓ a copy of the Resident's Bill of Rights must be posted in the resident's chart.

5. A violation of the resident's right to confidentiality would be

   Ⓐ discussing the resident's condition on a crowded elevator.
   Ⓑ discussing the resident's condition in a conference with nursing staff.
   Ⓒ writing the temperature of the resident on a scrap of paper.
   Ⓓ asking the nurse questions about the resident's condition.

6. What is your best response when a resident complains about the nursing home?

   Ⓐ Call the family and ask them to transfer the resident.
   Ⓑ Help the resident write a complaint letter.
   Ⓒ Listen closely to the resident and report the complaints to the nurse.
   Ⓓ Listen to the resident and explain there are things people can't change.

7. When a resident feels his or her rights have been infringed upon, he or she has the right to

   Ⓐ leave the facility without paying for care.
   Ⓑ remain in the facility without any additional cost.
   Ⓒ call the police or sheriff.
   Ⓓ file a grievance.

8. When preparing the resident to take part in activities, it is important to

   Ⓐ ask the resident which activity he or she would like to attend.
   Ⓑ take the resident to activities only after all your work is finished.
   Ⓒ take the resident to the activity of your choice so you can take part in the activity.
   Ⓓ wait for the family to take the resident to the activity.

9. You see another nursing assistant abusing a confused resident. What is your best response?

   Ⓐ Call the resident's family.
   Ⓑ Report this to your supervisor.
   Ⓒ Tell the other nursing assistant to stop that kind of behavior.
   Ⓓ Ignore it, since it is not your duty to watch other employees.

10. You can assist the resident in maintaining dignity and self-worth by

   Ⓐ letting him or her to make choices whenever possible.
   Ⓑ doing everything for each resident exactly the same.
   Ⓒ always calling the residents, "honey and dearie."
   Ⓓ doing things for the resident yourself to hurry and get done with your work.

11. Residents' possessions, such as photos and letters, should be

   Ⓐ placed in the facility's safe for safeguarding.
   Ⓑ sent home with the family.
   Ⓒ respected and handled with care.
   Ⓓ put away in closets at the nurse's station.

12. The Resident's Bill of Rights

   Ⓐ is a law for the doctors to follow.
   Ⓑ must be respected by all members of the health care facility.
   Ⓒ is a guideline for states to follow in providing services to residents.
   Ⓓ provides an outline of costs of care in long-term care facilities.

13. What should you do when tidying up a resident's room?

   Ⓐ Ask the resident before throwing away any articles.
   Ⓑ Bring all plants and flowers out of room.
   Ⓒ Throw out any newspapers or old magazines.
   Ⓓ Clean the room without telling resident.

14. When the resident exercises his or her right to refuse treatment,

   Ⓐ the resident must move out of the facility as soon as possible.
   Ⓑ the doctor and family must be called immediately in all cases.
   Ⓒ an explanation of the likely results of refusal of treatment must be given to the resident.
   Ⓓ the resident must inform the facility in writing before refusing treatment.

15. The resident's right to privacy would be violated if you

   Ⓐ opened his or her mail without the resident's permission.
   Ⓑ closed the door when taking the resident into the bathroom.
   Ⓒ pulled privacy curtains when giving care.
   Ⓓ exposed only necessary body parts when giving care to the resident

16. A resident asks for help to go to the facility gift shop to buy a teddy bear for a new grandchild. Your best response is

   Ⓐ "That teddy bear is expensive. How will you pay for it?"
   Ⓑ "It would be a waste of time. You don't have any money."
   Ⓒ "I'll try to take you after lunch or find someone who can."
   Ⓓ "Does your doctor know about this?"

ANSWERS

1. B	6. C	12. B
2. C	7. D	13. A
3. D	8. A	14. C
4. C	9. B	15. A
5. A	10. A	16. C
	11. C	

Chapter 4

Mental Health and Social Needs

In this chapter you will learn how you can help residents meet their mental health and social needs. After reading this chapter you should be able to:

- Define Key Terms
- Identify Characteristics of Residents with Mental Health Needs
- Describe Considerations to be Given to the Mentally Impaired Resident
- Describe Techniques of Behavior Management
- List Guidelines for Interacting with Residents Having Some Mental Impairment
- Describe Ways to Modify Your Behavior in Response to the Resident's Behavior

Key Terms

Alzheimer's disease: A disease of unknown cause resulting in gradual loss of mental abilities. This irreversible disease may take from a few months to years to progress to the stage of complete helplessness in individuals

Confusion: Behavior that is different from the usual and accepted; being mixed up

Dementia: Impairment of mental capabilities

Disorientation: Loss of or confusion about one's identity, the place or time

Lethargy: Abnormal drowsiness

Mental illness: A disorder of the mind

Mental retardation: Lower than average intellectual development; can range from mild to severe

Psychosocial needs: Those needs that have to do with mental and emotional activity

Reality orientation: A program designed to assist one to relearn dates, time, place, and identity

Characteristics of Residents With Mental Health Needs

Many residents in long-term care facilities need some help in meeting their **psychosocial needs**; however, some population groups have special mental health care needs. You will be caring for some residents who have mental disease. These residents may need physical care, but they will also need extra help in meeting their mental health needs. Knowing the possible mental impairments will help you care for these residents. Residents with **mental illness**, **mental retardation**, **Alzheimer's disease,** and other mental disorders will need special help from you.

Mental Orientation

Residents with mental impairments often are disoriented. That is, they are confused about where they are and the existing situation. Generally it is a frightening experience to feel disoriented. Understanding this feeling in yourself will help you to relate to the disoriented resident. An explanation of orientation follows:

○ Orientation is knowing
  • Who you are
  • Where you are
  • Who the persons around you are
  • The time (year, month, date, day of week, and time of day)

Population of the Long-Term Care Facility

Listed are some broad categories of mental health needs and characteristics of that resident who has the condition.

Residents with mental retardation

• Level of abilities varies among these residents

• Adjustment to new situations is often difficult

• These residents often have poor judgment and lack of foresight

• Socially inappropriate sexual behavior may occur

• Most residents have the ability to learn appropriate and necessary ADL skills with proper training, support, and guidance from a knowledgeable and caring staff

Residents with Mental Illness

- Changes in the personality of the mentally ill vary among residents and type of mental illness

- Medication, psychotherapy, and a supportive staff who have knowledge and understanding of behavior techniques can often help

- Common behaviors in mental illness include the following:

  - inappropriate social behavior
    - varies from not sleeping to talking excessively

  - unusual level of activity
    - varies from overactivity (pacing) to underactivity (refusing to move)

  - sleep disturbances
    - varies from excessive sleeping to having difficulty getting to sleep or awakening extremely early

  - delusions
    - having false beliefs

  - hallucinations
    - seeing, hearing, or smelling things that are not present

  - compulsive behaviors
    - performing a behavior over and over

  - anxiety

  - confusion

  - angry outbursts

  - weeping without cause

  - laughing without cause

  - fear

  - withdrawal

Residents with Alzheimer's Disease and Other Related Disorders

Alzheimer's disease is a form of dementia or mental illness of unknown cause. It creates changes in the brain tissue that ends up as gradual loss of mental abilities. **Dementia** is defined as the deterioration or decline of the brain or impairment of mental capabilities. Dementia can be caused by acute (over a short period) or chronic (over a long period) disease. Characteristics of Alzheimer's and other dementias vary with individuals and may include the following:

- Trouble sleeping

- Wandering or becoming confused in the evening

- Poor memory of recent past

- Memory of long past is often very clear

- Lack of orientation to time and place

- Asking the same questions

- Creating new words

- Misidentifying people

- Lethargy or restlessness

- Becoming easily agitated and cannot be calmed readily

- Problems with movement

- Incontinence of bowel or bladder

The above symptoms may increase in severity to the point where the resident needs help in all activities of daily living.

Considerations for the Mentally Impaired Resident

The mentally impaired resident needs the same physical care as any other resident. Remember all people have the same basic physical and psychosocial needs. Be aware of these basic human needs as you care for the resident with Alzheimer's disease, dementia, or another mental impairment.

Special considerations necessary for the mentally impaired resident are the following:

- ○ Environment

  - Provide a structured safe environment

  - Avoid changes

  - Avoid excessive stimulation. Too much activity and noise often adds to confusion and anxiety

  - Avoid isolating the resident. Isolation leads to further confusion

  - Supervise wandering residents adequately

- ○ Oral communication

  - Call resident by preferred name. All staff members should be consistent

  - Use calm voice and speak softly

  - Keep communication simple. Give simple, short instructions

- Allow time for resident to respond

- Mention the resident's emotional feelings that are evident, such as fear or sadness

- **Reality orientation** should be practiced by all staff

  ○ Point to clocks and calendars. Use verbal orientation to time, place, day, date, etc

○ Body language

- Approach resident from the front (many persons with Alzheimer's disease have decreased ability to see side views)

- Face the resident. Make eye contact

- Bend down to same level as resident rather than standing over the resident when talking

- Use hand movements to enhance understanding

- Remain calm and reassuring

- Use calm body language. Avoid jerky, rapid body movements

- Use touch to reassure

○ Knowledge of resident's past

- Listen to the resident's family. They may be able to give suggestions or ideas that help you in the resident's care. Many families had been caring for the resident with mental illness for a long time at home.

- Ask the nurse or social worker for information

- Realize information about the resident is to be held in confidence

Behavior Management

All behavior has a meaning. It may mean one thing to the person exhibiting the behavior and something very different to the person observing the behavior. It is often difficult to understand the mentally impaired resident's behavior. To that resident, however, the behavior has a purpose. Many behaviors we see as problems are the result of fears and unmet needs. As a nursing assistant, you must be patient, respectful, and always treat each resident with dignity.

Many residents have lost some control over their life due to many types of disabilities. This loss of control causes inappropriate behavior. Offering choices whenever possible gives the resident a sense of control, which reduces frustration. Fewer frustrations will often result in fewer behavior problems (Figure 4-1).

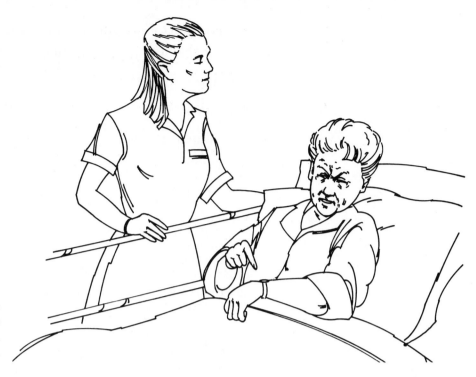

FIGURE 4-1.
Understanding the resident's
frustrations will help you deal
with the resident.

Techniques to Reinforce Appropriate Behavior

- Refer to care plan regarding special methods, techniques, or strategies

- Respond to appropriate behavior with genuine compliments and praise

- Show pleasant response at appropriate behavior by nonverbal communication, smiles, touch, etc.

- Show as little response as possible to inappropriate behavior

- Never laugh at or ridicule resident's behavior

- Remember that all behaviors have meaning to the person doing it

Guidelines for Interacting with Mentally Impaired Residents

This section has some general techniques to follow when interacting with residents having some mental impairment. Because each resident is an individual person, there may be special instructions and/or restrictions for certain residents.

The need for individualized care is essential. Be sure you follow any special instructions listed on the care plan. Consistency is very important when dealing with residents having mental impairment. Some general guidelines include the following:

- Become aware of your own responses and reactions to the resident's behavior and modify your behavior, if necessary

- Develop caring attitudes

  - patience

  - kindness

  - pleasantness

  - gentleness

  - caring

  - understanding

- Reinforce feelings of belonging and safety by saying such things as "You're safe here, " or "This is your home"

- Call the resident by the name they prefer

- Treat the resident with dignity and respect. Do not talk "down" to the resident, or treat him or her as a child. Never use any degrading names or terms

- Always be calm in verbal and nonverbal communication

- Avoid changes in the resident's environment. Maintain structure of daily routines

- Dress and groom the resident in appropriate attire

- To be consistent, report all successes and failures at attempts to modify resident behaviors

- Acknowledge the resident's feelings by saying such things as, "I can see you are afraid" or "I can see you're feeling sad"

- Help the resident have feelings of positive self-esteem. Behavior problems will decrease

- Allow the resident to do as much as possible. This increases feelings of self-worth

- Support the family members and listen to their suggestions. Tell them about activities where family involvement is encouraged

- Understand the resident. Think how you would like to be treated if you or your parent were the resident

Behavior Modifications for Nursing Assistants

This section has some specific ways you as a nursing assistant can change your behavior in response to the resident. These techniques can help you when working with a resident having mental impairment.

○ Demonstrate Body Language that Communicates a Listening Approach toward Resident

- Place yourself near resident but show respect for the resident's "personal space"

- Position yourself at resident's level. Sit if resident is sitting; stand if resident is standing

- Face the resident

- Assume open posture, by avoiding crossed arms and legs

- Lean toward resident

- Make eye contact

- Appear relaxed, and avoid fidgeting or looking around

- Use nonverbal behavior to express interest in what the resident is saying, by smiling, nodding head, raising eyebrows, etc.

- Report or record the resident's behavior and responses to your behavior

○ Manage and Decrease Aggressive or Agitated Behavior of Resident

- Base actions on principle that anger is a secondary emotional response to a primary feeling of fear, frustration, grief, or loss of self-esteem

- If no risk to yourself or others exists, ignore the resident's behavior

- Approach the resident from the front

- Move slowly and deliberately

- Make eye contact

- Speak with a low-pitched voice in a calm, firm manner

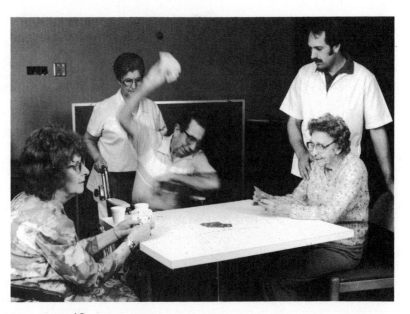

FIGURE 4-2.
Protect other residents when a resident is showing his anger.

- Speak in short, simple phrases
- Acknowledge feelings that are evident by saying, "I can see you are angry," or "I can see you are frightened"
- Be sure to tell the resident he or she is safe
- Allow resident to talk about his or her anger
- Listen to the resident
- If possible, use the resident's anger constructively by getting them to do such things as wiping a table, tearing rags, squeezing a ball, or rolling a ball of yarn
- Use isolation and restraints only when necessary and as indicated on the care plan (Figure 4-2)
- Report or record resident's behavior and responses to your behavior

Key Points in This Chapter

🔑 Residents with mental impairments will need special assistance in meeting their psychosocial needs.

🔑 Symptoms of mental impairment vary according to the disease.

🔑 Special consideration must be given to the mentally impaired resident.

🔑 Alzheimer's disease is a form of dementia resulting in gradual loss of mental abilities.

🔑 All behavior has some meaning to the person doing it.

🔑 Inappropriate behavior often is caused by feelings of loss of control over one's life.

🔑 Offering choices and allowing residents to do as much as possible gives them some sense of control and adds to feelings of self-esteem.

🔑 Consistency in care is extremely important for the resident with mental impairment.

Review Quiz Chapter 4
Mental Health and Social Needs

Choose the best answer for the questions below.

1. A resident who is disoriented is

    (A) usually retarded.
    (B) confused as to time and place.
    (C) not allowed to eat.
    (D) also destructive.

2. Changes in the personality of a resident is often a sign of

    (A) some degree of mental illness.
    (B) unmet physical needs.
    (C) too much socializing.
    (D) lack of exercise.

3. Alzheimer's disease creates changes in the

    (A) kidneys.
    (B) heart.
    (C) lungs.
    (D) brain.

4. A resident with dementia needs

    (A) increased activity to stay alert.
    (B) to be isolated from others.
    (C) a structured, safe environment.
    (D) freedom from rules.

5. In understanding what kind of meaning a particular behavior has, it is important to know that all behavior has the most meaning and purpose to

    (A) the facility psychologist.
    (B) the person doing the behavior.
    (C) the person watching the behavior.
    (D) the person who is talking.

6. Inappropriate behavior by residents is often caused by

    (A) activity.
    (B) isolation.
    (C) confidence.
    (D) frustration.

7. When speaking to residents, call them

    (A) granny or gramps.
    (B) the name they prefer.
    (C) a friendly nickname.
    (D) "honey" or "dear."

8. When residents have feelings of positive self-esteem, behavior problems

    (A) are decreased.
    (B) are increased.
    (C) stay the same.
    (D) get started.

9. When taking care of residents with a mental impairment, you should keep their daily routine

    (A) full of recreational activities.
    (B) varied so they don't get bored.
    (C) the same from day to day.
    (D) free of any exercise.

10. To build feelings of self-esteem in residents with mental illness

    (A) do things for them quickly so they don't have to wait.
    (B) tell them what clothing looks best on them.
    (C) allow them to do as much as possible for themselves.
    (D) always feed them so they don't spill food.

11. When you *empathize* with the resident, you are feeling

  Ⓐ like you think they feel.
  Ⓑ very badly for them.
  Ⓒ very sorry for them.
  Ⓓ very happy for them.

12. A good listening approach to use when working with a resident with a mental impairment is to

  Ⓐ tell the resident to stop talking.
  Ⓑ keep some distance between yourself and the resident.
  Ⓒ sit down by the resident who is in a chair.
  Ⓓ never look the resident in the eye.

13. When a resident is angry or agitated, the underlying emotion is usually

  Ⓐ fear.
  Ⓑ love.
  Ⓒ hate.
  Ⓓ depression.

14. A resident seems very angry and announces "No one is going to tell me what to do!" Your best response is

  Ⓐ immediately apply a restraint.
  Ⓑ allow the resident to verbalize anger.
  Ⓒ tell the resident to "cool it."
  Ⓓ give the resident a hug.

15. A good example of providing choices to a resident would be to

  Ⓐ tell the resident to go for a walk outside.
  Ⓑ allow resident to choose a dessert providing all of dinner is eaten first.
  Ⓒ allow resident to pick out clothes to wear today.
  Ⓓ explain that if he or she chooses to be angry, there will be no bingo games.

ANSWERS
1. B
2. A
3. D
4. C
5. B
6. D
7. B
8. A
9. C
10. C
11. A
12. C
13. A
14. B
15. C

Chapter 5

Communication

In this chapter you will learn the importance of communication with the residents and between members of the health care team in the long-term care facility. After reading this chapter you should be able to:

- Define Key Terms
- Define Effective Communication
- Identify Types of Communication
- List Characteristics of Therapeutic Communication
- Describe Barriers to Communication
- Describe the Importance of Communication with Staff
- List Examples of Observations to be Reported
- Describe the Nursing Assistant's Role in Record Keeping
- Identify Common Medical Abbreviations

Key Terms

Barrier: A barricade; something that hinders or separates

Communication: The exchange of thoughts, feelings, and information by verbal or nonverbal messages

Legible: Plain, easily read

Medical record: The resident's chart; the written legal record of the history and progress of the resident

Nonverbal: Sending a message without the use of words; body language

Observation: Noticing a fact or occurrences

Therapeutic: Serving to cure, heal, or preserve health

Verbal: Sending a message by using words and voice

Effective **communication** is essential in your role as a nursing assistant. In order to do you job well in the long-term care facility, you must develop good comunication skills for relating to the residents, their family members and visitors, and the staff (Fighure 5-1). Communication includes three things:

A sender
A message
A receiver

Effective communication occurs when the receiver gets the message in the way the sender meant the message. To communicate well takes time, practice, and skill. Since you will be spending a lot of your working day with individual residents, you have a responsibility to encourage the resident to talk about his needs. Using the techniques listed will help encourage residents to verbalize (talk about) needs. Guidelines for effective communication are the following:

• Reduce background noise (music, television)

• Make sure your body language says you are listening

• Speak at a pace the resident understands

• Give the resident time to talk

• Express an interest in what the resident says

• Make eye contact

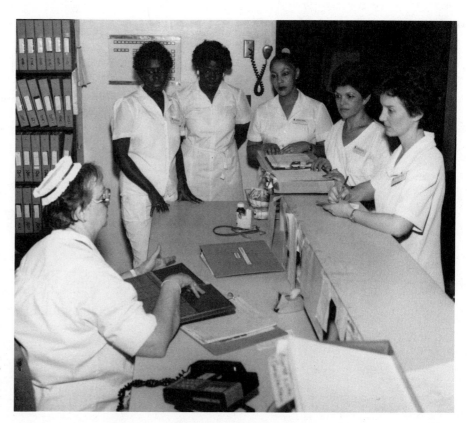

FIGURE 5-1.
Communication with other staff members is essential for nursing assistants.

- Match body language with what is said

- Speak clearly and at an appropriate noise level for resident to be able to hear you

- Refer to resident by the name the resident prefers

Types of Communication

Communication occurs in two ways: **verbal** or **nonverbal**. You will use both forms of communication as you work with residents. Some important points about verbal and nonverbal communication are the following:

Verbal Communication

- Get the message across through the use of voice or words

- Use it to give and receive information, to report facts, and to share experiences

- Verbal communication consists of

  - choice of words

  - tone of voice

  - speed of voice

- Be alert to the resident's ability to understand the words you use

Nonverbal Communication

- Get a message across without the use of words

- Examples of nonverbal communication include facial expressions, posture, hand gestures, touch, dress, movements, raising of eyebrows, smiling, frowns, silence, etc.

- Remember that actions speak louder than words. Be aware of your nonverbal behavior when relating to the resident and his or her family or visitors

Therapeutic Communication

The words therapy and **therapeutic** mean healing or improving a situation. Therapeutic communication can be either verbal or nonverbal. You have probably used therapeutic communication quite often. For example, how often have you felt better after talking something over with someone or helping a friend through a sad situation by just being there? As a nursing assistant, you will be in a position to provide therapeutic communication for the resident. Successful therapeutic communication is possible only if you understand what the resident is really trying to tell you (Figure 5-2). Some points to remember are the following:

- Listen carefully to what the resident is saying

- Observe the resident's movements and actions

- Be sensitive to the resident's feelings. Notice any differences between the words and actions

- Comment on the resident's feelings by giving appropriate responses

- Provide feedback so both you and the resident understand what was communicated

- Report to the nurse the resident's responses, actions, and behaviors

Communication Barriers

Anything that interferes with the communication process can be considered a **barrier**, something that makes communication difficult. The barrier can be from either the sender or receiver and can interfere during any part of communication. Also, both verbal and nonverbal barriers can occur. Some barriers to effective communication are the following:

- Not listening

- Background noise

- Belittling a person

- Talking to a resident as you would a child

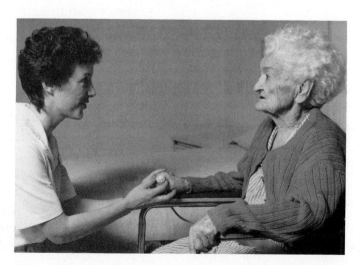

FIGURE 5-2.
Take time to talk to the resident.

- Taking over the conversation

- Avoiding eye contact

- Appearing too busy or in a hurry

- Making judgments

- Not acknowledging what was said

- Giving false or inappropriate answers

- Using words the resident does not understand

- Physical disability such as impaired vision, hearing or ability to speak

Communication with the Vision-impaired Resident

Since some vision loss is part of the normal aging process, you will be working with vision-impaired residents. This vision impairment often is a barrier to communicating with the elderly resident. The resident's care plan will identify specific methods for assisting the resident.

Common techniques to use are the following:

- Identify yourself when approaching resident

- Knock before entering room

- Call the resident by the name he or she wishes to be called

- Recognize that the glare from window behind you can interfere with resident's ability to see clearly

- Encourage use of and help resident with eyeglasses. Making sure eyeglasses are clean

- Explain where items are. Keep them in the same place so environment is familiar

- Offer your arm to guide the resident. Walk slightly ahead of resident

- Speak clearly and slowly using moderate tone of voice

- Do not talk to resident as if he or she is a child

Communication with the Hearing-impaired Resident

Some hearing loss occurs in the normal aging process. Hearing loss can be a severe barrier to communicating with the resident. Specific suggestions will be listed on the resident's care plan.

Common techniques to use are the following:

- Identify yourself to the resident

- Gently touch the resident to get attention

- Face the resident when talking

- Speak clearly and slowly

- Keep hands away from your face while talking

- Stand or sit near the resident

- Do not eat or chew while talking to the resident

- If the resident uses a hearing aid, help insert it (Figure 5-3)

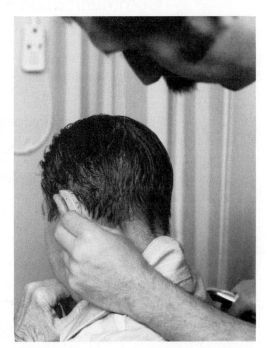

FIGURE 5-3.
Parts of a hearing aid.

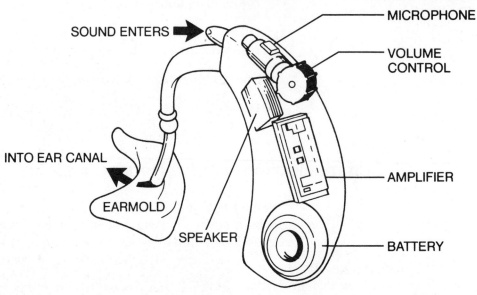

SOUND ENTERS ➡️

MICROPHONE

VOLUME CONTROL

INTO EAR CANAL

AMPLIFIER

EARMOLD

SPEAKER

BATTERY

Communication With Staff

Because nursing assistants have frequent and close contact with the resident, you will have the opportunity to observe the resident more closely than the supervising nurse. Communicating with the nurse about the resident is absolutely necessary for continuity of care (Figure 5-4).

The care plan is an essential tool for staff communication regarding the resident's care. The care plan is a written plan that clearly identifies a resident's needs. Your responsibilities for the resident's care are listed on the care plan. Your supervising nurse will help you develop your assignment based on information in the care plan. You should ask the nurse any questions when you are given your assignment. Your supervising nurse will help you determine how to prioritize (arrange) your assignment. Remember, the Resident's Bill of Rights gives the resident the right to have privacy regarding his medical records. Be sure you discuss the resident's condition in a private setting with the nurse.

Reporting Observations

Because of your close contact with the resident, you must know what must be reported to the nurse. Certain **observations** must be reported immediately. If there is any doubt in your mind, it is always best to report any change to the nurse right away.

Some guidelines on what to observe and report are the following:

- Any change in the resident's physical or mental status

- Resident's reactions and behaviors

- What the resident says about his or her health (i.e., pain, numbness, dizziness)

- Care that seems to work best for the resident

- What care does not seem to work well

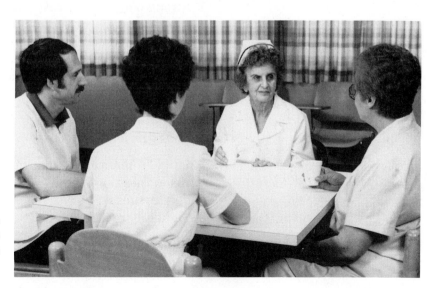

FIGURE 5-4.
The nursing assistant works with other members of the health care team.

How to Recognize and Report Abnormal Signs and Symptoms

The following are signs and symptoms that tell you something is not normal. They may indicate disease or illness in the resident and must be brought to the nurse's attention.

- Any evidence of pain
  - in chest
  - when moving
  - while urinating
  - while having a bowel movement

- Skin changes
  - any redness
  - breaks or tears
  - bruises
  - lumps
  - abnormal sweating
  - swelling (feet, ankles, and hands)
  - skin feels very warm or cool
  - bluish color in lips or fingertips

- Respiratory changes
  - coughing
  - rapid breathing
  - shortness of breath
  - noisy breathing

- Digestive changes
  - nausea
  - vomiting
  - appetite changes
  - excessive thirst
  - difficulty in swallowing or chewing
  - dark or bloody stool
  - watery or hard stool

- Urinary changes
  - difficulty urinating
  - dark color
  - strong odor
  - blood, mucous, or sediment in urine
  - urinating in small amounts
  - burning or pain while urinating
  - suddenly cannot control passage of urine

- Musculoskeletal changes
  - cannot move arms or legs
  - shaky or jerky motions

- Change in mental status
  - drowsiness
  - restlessness
  - suddenly more confused
  - problem with coordination

○ Other changes
  • fever or chills
  • any unusual body discharge (pus, mucous)

Record Keeping

The resident's **medical record** is often called the resident's chart. This is a legal document that contains the history and progress of the resident's care in the health care facility. Record-keeping policies, or charting, are not the same at all facilities. In many facilities, the nursing assistant is responsible for some of the important record keeping. Patterns of or changes in the resident's behavior are noticed because of the nursing assistant's reporting and recording. Most facilities require nursing assistants to do checklist charting. Examples of checklist charting are the following:

• ADL (activities of daily living) sheets

• bowel sheets

• I&O (Intake and Output) sheets

• Meal sheets

• TPR (temperature, pulse, and respiration) & BP (blood pressure) sheets

Charting must be accurate, clearly written, **legible**, confidential, dated, and signed (Figure 5-5).

Medical Abbreviations

You must know some commonly used medical abbreviations to communicate well with the nursing staff.

Become familiar with the following abbreviations:

$\bar{c}$ — with

$\bar{s}$ — without

q — every

q. d. — every day

q. o. d. — every other day

b. i. d. — twice a day

t. i. d. — three times a day

q. i. d. — four times a day

ADL — activities of daily living

ad lib — as desired

Amb. — ambulate, to walk

B&B — bowel and bladder program

BM — bowel movement

BP — blood pressure

HS — hour of sleep (bedtime)

I&O — intake and output

NPO — nothing by mouth

O_2 — oxygen

PRN, prn — whenever necessary

PROM — Passive range of motion

Stat — at once

S&A — sugar and acetone

TPR — temperature, pulse, respiration

VS — vital signs

W/C — wheelchair

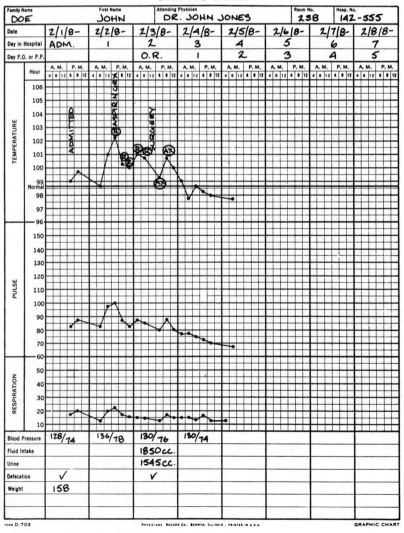

FIGURE 5-5.
A sample of a TPR and BP sheet.

Key Points in This Chapter

- Effective communication occurs when the message received is the same as the one sent.

- Communication can be either verbal or nonverbal.

- A barrier to communication is anything that blocks communication.

- Common barriers to effective communication with the elderly resident are vision, hearing, and speech impairments.

- The nursing assistant has the most opportunities in the long-term care facility to observe the resident. Reporting these observations to the nurse is an important role of the nursing assistant.

- Any record keeping must be accurate, legible, confidential. It must also be signed by the person doing the recording.

- Medical abbreviations are used in the health care setting to help you communicate well.

Review Quiz Chapter 5
Communication

Choose the best answer for the questions below.

1. Communication is said to be effective when

    Ⓐ message is sent correctly.

    Ⓑ message is received as sender wants it to be received.

    Ⓒ message is received as receiver wants to receive the message.

    Ⓓ message is sent as sender intends but received differently.

2. Which of the following are included as techniques in good communication?

    Ⓐ Speak clearly and loud enough for resident to hear.

    Ⓑ Reduce background noise.

    Ⓒ Avoid looking at resident while talking.

    Ⓓ All of the above.

    Ⓔ A and B only.

3. Verbal communication is

    Ⓐ sending a message using words.

    Ⓑ using touch to send a message.

    Ⓒ the same as nonverbal communication.

    Ⓓ sending a message without the use of words.

4. When communication is performed with an idea of improving a situation, it is called

    Ⓐ improved communication.

    Ⓑ therapeutic communication.

    Ⓒ medical communication.

    Ⓓ verbal communication.

5. What is an example of a communication barrier?

    Ⓐ Listening attentively

    Ⓑ Observing the facial expression

    Ⓒ Maintaining eye contact

    Ⓓ Talking "down" to a person, as to a child

6. When communicating with the resident who has a vision impairment, it is important to

    Ⓐ speak louder than usual.

    Ⓑ encourage the resident to wear his or her glasses.

    Ⓒ give the resident written instructions instead of saying them.

    Ⓓ keep resident's room as dark as possible to eliminate eye strain.

7. Communication with a resident who has a hearing impairment may be improved by

    Ⓐ facing the resident when talking.

    Ⓑ standing or sitting close to the resident when talking.

    Ⓒ assisting the resident with the use of the hearing aid.

    Ⓓ All of the above

8. What member of the nursing staff often has the most frequent contact with the resident?

    Ⓐ The head nurse

    Ⓑ The team leader

    Ⓒ The medication nurse

    Ⓓ The nursing assistant

9. The essential tool in staff communication regarding the resident's care is the

Ⓐ care plan.
Ⓑ team report.
Ⓒ medical report.
Ⓓ assignment sheet.

10. Which of the following are important for you to report to the nurse?

Ⓐ Gifts brought to the resident
Ⓑ The television shows the resident watches
Ⓒ Any change in the resident's physical status or health
Ⓓ All of the above

11. When observing *skin* changes in the resident, you should notice and report

Ⓐ shortness of breath.
Ⓑ redness or swelling.
Ⓒ digestive disturbances.
Ⓓ drowsiness or restlessness.

12. The legal document that contains the resident's medical history and progress is

Ⓐ the care plan.
Ⓑ the medical chart.
Ⓒ the assignment sheet.
Ⓓ the Medicare report.

13. All of the following are true about recording (charting) on the medical record *except*

Ⓐ charting must be accurate.
Ⓑ charting must be clearly written.
Ⓒ no signature is required on any charting.
Ⓓ the information on the medical record is confidential.

14. Medical terms and abbreviations are used in the health care setting to

Ⓐ encourage staff to learn new words.
Ⓑ discourage residents from understanding medical findings.
Ⓒ keep information in code in case it is overheard by visitors.
Ⓓ assist in making staff communication clear and concise.

15. What does B.P. at H.S. mean?

Ⓐ Give bedpan at his/her side
Ⓑ Give bedpan at hour of sleep
Ⓒ Take blood pressure at bedtime
Ⓓ Take blood pressure at his/her side

16. The abbreviation for three times a day is

Ⓐ 3xd
Ⓑ t. i. d.
Ⓒ 3 i. d.
Ⓓ t. o. d.

17. Abnormal digestive changes that you should recognize and report are

Ⓐ swollen ankles.
Ⓑ shortness of breath.
Ⓒ dark or hard stools.
Ⓓ pain while urinating.

Chapter 6

Infection Control

In this chapter you will learn the principles of infection control. You must understand these principles to prevent the spread of disease in the health care setting. After reading this chapter you should be able to:

- Define Key Terms
- List Principles of Medical Asepsis
- Define Infection
- Describe Universal Precautions
- Demonstrate Proper Hand Washing
- Perform Isolation Procedures

Key Terms

Aseptic: The absence of any disease-causing microbes

Bacteria: One-celled microorganisms, some of which cause disease

Communicable: Diseases that are easily transmitted to other persons

Contaminate: To become unclean, soiled

Disinfection: The process that destroys disease-causing microorganisms and slows down growth of others

Germs: A common name for disease-causing microbes

Infection: A disease state caused by microorganisms invading the body

Isolation: Techniques involved in caring for the person with a communicable disease

Medical asepsis: The practices and techniques used in the medical setting to prevent the spread of microorganisms from one person or place to another. Sometimes called *Clean Technique*

Microbe: A microorganism

Microorganism: Living plants and animals that are so small they can only be seen with a microscope

Pathogen: A microorganism that is harmful and causes disease; disease-causing microbes

Sterile: The absence of all microorganisms, i. e., those causing disease and those that do not

Sterilization: The process that destroys all microorganisms

Universal precautions: Special procedures and practices taken when working with people or items contaminated with specific diseases

Virus: Extremely small microbes that grow on living plants and animals

Medical Asepsis

Medical asepsis means practices and techniques used in the health care facility to prevent the spread of disease. **Aseptic** means to be free from disease-causing microorganisms. The staff in a health care facility must use the principles of medical asepsis to prevent the spread of diseases (Figure 6-1). An understanding of microorganisms will help you to realize the importance of medical asepsis.

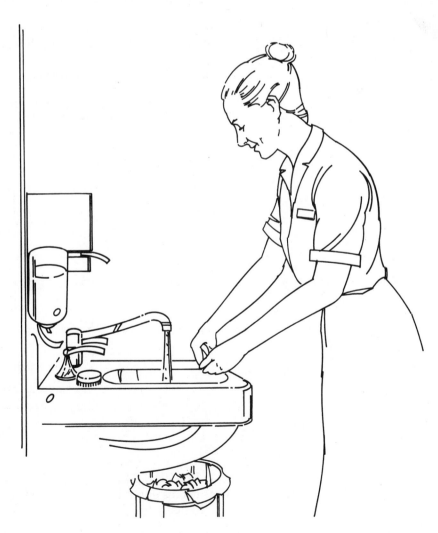

FIGURE 6-1.
Proper hand washing is important
for the nursing assistant.

Microorganisms

Microorganisms are small, living plants and animals that cannot be seen without using a microscope. Microorganisms, also called **microbes**, are found everywhere. They are in the air, in soil, in water, on food, on clothing, and on our body. Microbes need food, warmth, and moisture to grow and thrive. They grow best in a warm, dark, damp area. Microorganisms do not grow as well in light and dry areas. Disease-causing microbes are called **pathogens**. Pathogens can be destroyed by **disinfection**. **Sterilization** is required to kill all microorganisms.

In the long-term care facility, all persons are exposed to many microorganisms. Using the principles of medical asepsis in the long-term care facility is very important. Many of the residents do not have strong resistance to disease. In other words, their bodies cannot fight disease. In the health care facility you must prevent the spread of disease from resident to resident, resident to staff, or staff to resident (Figure 6-2).

Practices of Medical Asepsis

Principles of medical asepsis include the following:

○ Hand washing, which is the single most important measure in prevention of spreading of disease

○ Separation of clean and dirty items

○ Disinfection of supplies and equipment

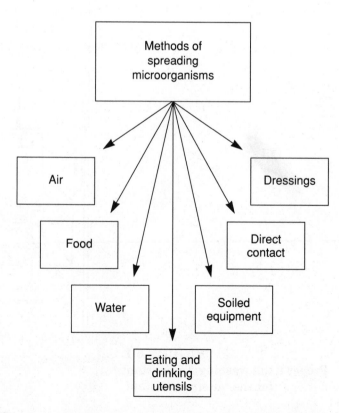

FIGURE 6-2.
Microorganisms can be spread in many ways.

- Proper handling of food

- Proper handling of linens
  - Do not have linen touch uniform
  - Do not place soiled linen on the floor
  - Avoid shaking of linens
  - If linen falls to floor, place it in soiled linen hamper
  - Grossly soiled linen must be pre-rinsed before placing in linen hamper

- Dispose of soiled liquids directly into sinks or toilets. Avoid splashing

- Proper handling of body waste
  - Dispose of wastes properly
  - Follow facility policy

- Maintain your own good health
  - Eat properly
  - Get enough sleep
  - Get adequate exercise
  - Maintain good mental health

- Staff and visitors should stay away from facility when they are ill

- Remember that hand washing is the single most effective way to prevent the spread of disease

Infection

An **infection** is a disease state that results from the invasion and growth of microorganisms (germs) in the body. The infection may be localized—confined to a certain body part or body area. Or the infection may be generalized— involving the whole body.

Development of Infection

Developing an infection is dependent on the following factors:

source: A germ that causes the disease

reservoir or host: A place where the source or germ can grow

carrier: A reservoir or host (usually a person) who may or may not have the signs of disease

transmission: Some way for the germ to get from the reservoir or host to another host

portal of entry: A place where the germ can get into the host body

susceptibility: The ability of the host body to resist the disease-causing germ

Disease Resistance

Knowing how infection develops is important for you to know, because you will be working with people who get ill very easily. A person's ability to resist infection and illness is related to the following:

- age

- general health and nutritional state

- medications taken by the person

- presence of other illness

Universal Precautions

Universal precautions are special procedures developed to protect you from disease when handling body discharges. Universal precautions require that all health care workers routinely use appropriate techniques when exposed to blood or body fluids. A health care facility may develop specific policies, but most generally include the following:

- Wear gloves when in contact with body fluids or body discharges such as:
  - blood
  - stool
  - urine
  - saliva
  - sputum
  - wound drainage
  - any other body fluids

- Change gloves after contact with each resident

- Wash hands after removing gloves

- Have gloves with you at all times

- Wear gloves, gown, mask, and cap when indicated. Isolation procedure follows later in this chapter

- Dispose of trash and linen properly. Place in sturdy plastic bag, do not allow soiled material to touch outside of bag

- Laundry and trash bags should be labeled as contaminated or as indicated by facility policy

- Follow procedure of facility regarding special situations

- Needles must be thrown away in special containers

- If you find a soiled or used needle, follow directions of supervisor for throwing it away

Hand Washing

As you have learned, hand washing is the single most effective way to prevent the spread of disease. Hand washing should be done

- When beginning work

- Before and after caring for each resident

- Before handling food

- After using the bathroom

- After combing your hair, using a tissue, eating, drinking or smoking

- After handling a resident's belongings

- After working with anything soiled

- After removing gloves

Other guidelines (Figure 6-3) to follow when washing your hands are the following:

- Use warm, running water

- Do not lean against the sink when washing. The sink is considered *contaminated*

- Avoid shaking water from your hands. Shaking water may spread the microbes

- Friction is required in hand washing. Friction is created by rubbing the hands together briskly. It is the friction that removes the germs from the hands

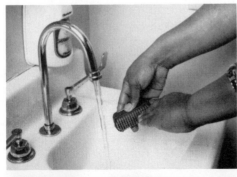
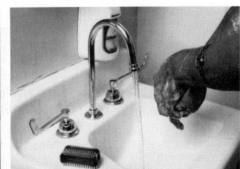
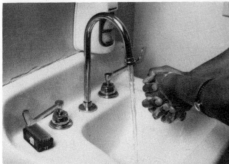
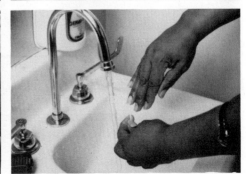

FIGURE 6-3.
Hand washing is the single most effective way to prevent the spread of disease.

- Dry your hands thoroughly

- Lotion your hands frequently. Frequent washing tends to dry out hands

- Follow facility policy for use of soap or other hand-cleaning agents

Procedure 2

Hand Washing

1. Stand away from sink. Uniform and hands must not touch sink.

2. Turn on water, using a paper towel, adjust water to warm, comfortable temperature.

3. Wet hands and wrists.

4. Apply soap over hands and wrists working into a lather.

5. Use friction when washing hands, fingers, and wrists.

6. Wash for one minute.

7. Rinse hands and wrists under running water.

8. Do not shake water from hands.

9. Dry hands and wrists with clean paper towel.

10. Turn off faucets, using clean paper towel.

11. Throw away paper towel.

(See Procedure Review, page 205)

Isolation Procedures

Isolation is a method or technique of caring for residents who have **communicable** or contagious diseases. The purpose of isolation is to prevent the spread of the disease.

The procedures in isolation vary with the disease. Many facilities use a color coded system that tells you which procedure to follow. Most isolation procedures include wearing a gown, gloves, and a mask (Figure 6-4). Knowing this procedure will help you stay healthy, and prevent the spread of disease.

Procedure 3

Isolation Procedures

A. Procedure for gowning, gloving, and masking using disposable gown, gloves, and mask

1. Remove your jewelry.

2. Wash your hands and dry them thoroughly.

3. Put on mask, adjust over nose and mouth, and tie securely at back of head.

4. Put on gown, making certain gown overlaps in back covering all clothing.

5. Tie neck ties.

6. Tie waist ties, making certain gown is overlapping.

7. Put on gloves covering cuff of gown with top edge of glove.

B. Procedure for removal

1. Make sure that all jobs in isolation unit are completed and that the resident is comfortable and safe.

2. Untie waist ties and tie in front of gown. This prevents contaminated ties from touching your uniform.

3. Remove first glove by grasping cuff of glove and pulling off. Throw away in trash container.

4. Remove second glove by placing bare hand inside the cuff of glove and pulling it off. Throw away in trash container.

5. Grasp the neck ties of the gown and untie. The neck ties are considered a clean area.

6. Loosen the gown at the shoulders, touching only the inside of the gown.

7. Slip fingers of one hand under cuff of gown at opposite arm. Do not touch outside of gown. Pull it down over hand.

8. With hand inside of gown, pull gown off of other arm.

9. Fold and roll gown with the contaminated side in.

10. Throw away in trash container.

11. Remove mask by grasping only the ties.

12. Throw away mask in trash container.

13. Use paper towel to turn on faucets.

14. Wash hands.

15. Open door with paper towel.

16. Repeat hand washing or use disinfectant as policy of your facility indicates.

(See Procedure Review, page 207)

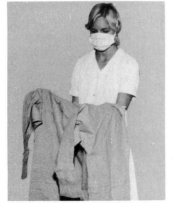 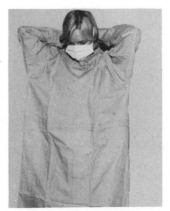 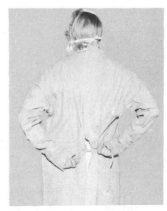

FIGURE 6-4a-c. If gowning is required, follow facility policy.

Key Points in This Chapter

🔑 Medical asepsis refers to practices performed to prevent the spread of disease.

🔑 Microorganisms are found everywhere. Many are present on the body.

🔑 Microorganisms live well in warm, dark, damp areas.

🔑 Most residents in the long-term care facility have lower resistance to disease, which means most are more susceptible to illness.

🔑 Proper hand washing is the single most effective way to prevent the spread of disease.

🔑 Friction is required when washing hands.

🔑 Infections can be localized or generalized.

🔑 Universal precautions are special procedures to be used when handling any body fluids.

🔑 Isolation procedures may be necessary to prevent the spread of communicable diseases.

Review Quiz Chapter 6
Infection Control

Choose the best answer for the questions below.

1. Practices used in health care facilities to prevent the spread of disease are referred to as

   Ⓐ sterilization.
   Ⓑ disinfection.
   Ⓒ medical asepsis.
   Ⓓ techniques.

2. Which of the following is *not* true regarding microorganisms?

   Ⓐ All microorganisms are harmful to humans.
   Ⓑ Microorganisms are small, living plants or animals.
   Ⓒ Microorganisms need food, warmth and moisture to grow.
   Ⓓ Microorganisms are present in many places.

3. What is the *most* important measure nursing assistants can do to prevent the spread of disease?

   Ⓐ Sterilize all items.
   Ⓑ Wear isolation gowns.
   Ⓒ Wash hands.
   Ⓓ Wear gloves.

4. Proper handling of linens includes

   Ⓐ holding linens away from uniform.
   Ⓑ pre-rinse grossly soiled linen
   Ⓒ shake all linen vigorously.
   Ⓓ All of the above
   Ⓔ A and B only.

5. Microorganisms can be spread by all of the following *except*

   Ⓐ contaminated dressings.
   Ⓑ food and water.
   Ⓒ sterile items.
   Ⓓ the air.

6. A germ or microorganism that causes a disease is the

   Ⓐ carrier of disease.
   Ⓑ source of disease.
   Ⓒ host or reservoir.
   Ⓓ portal of entry.

7. Susceptibility to disease is affected by

   Ⓐ age.
   Ⓑ general health
   Ⓒ nutritional state.
   Ⓓ All of the above
   Ⓔ A and B only.

8. Special procedures developed to protect the worker from disease when handling body discharges are called

   Ⓐ discharge directions.
   Ⓑ waste disposal.
   Ⓒ universal precautions.
   Ⓓ precautions for disposal.

9. When wearing gloves, it is important to remember

   Ⓐ to wash hands after removing gloves.
   Ⓑ to change gloves at the end of shift only.
   Ⓒ to wash hands with gloves on between residents.
   Ⓓ there is no need to wash hands if you wear gloves.

10. Friction in hand washing is created by

   (A) lotion applied to hands.
   (B) rubbing the hands briskly.
   (C) using a mild soap.
   (D) warm water.

11. When washing your hands, use

   (A) a basin to soak hands.
   (B) cold water to slow germ growth.
   (C) warm running water.
   (D) as hot water as possible.

12. Which of the following is *not* correct when washing your hands?

   (A) Dry hands thoroughly.
   (B) Avoid shaking water from hands.
   (C) Work soap into a lather when washing.
   (D) Lean against the sink when washing hands.

13. After washing your hands, turn the faucet off

   (A) using a clean paper towel.
   (B) using a wet towel to clean the faucet.
   (C) with the same towel used to dry hands.
   (D) without a paper towel.

14. Proper hand washing for the nursing assistant includes washing

   (A) the hands only.
   (B) the hands and wrists.
   (C) the hands, wrists, and arms up to the elbows.
   (D) only the hand that touched something contaminated.

15. A disease state caused by invasion of microorganisms into the body that can be either localized or generalized is a(n)

   (A) invasion.
   (B) disability.
   (C) infection.
   (D) germ.

16. Microorganisms live best in

   (A) very dry areas.
   (B) dark, damp, warm areas.
   (C) sunlight areas.
   (D) cold, wet areas.

17. If a resident has an infected hand, it would be an example of a

   (A) generalized infection.
   (B) transmission infection.
   (C) process infection.
   (D) localized infection.

18. Microorganisms that are harmful and cause disease are called

   (A) toxins.
   (B) pathogens.
   (C) disinfections.
   (D) aseptics.

Chapter 7

Comfort, Safety, and Emergency Measures

In this chapter you will learn safety and emergency measures you need to know when working in a long-term care facility. After reading this chapter you should be able to:

- Define Key Terms
- List Appropriate Safety Measures for Residents
- Apply a Vest Restraint
- Describe Your Role in Fire Safety Measures
- Demonstrate Principles of Body Mechanics
- Care for the Resident's Unit
- Make the Unoccupied Bed
- Identify Situations that call for Emergency Action

Key Terms

Body mechanics: Special ways of standing and moving one's body to make best use of strength and to avoid fatigue

Cardiopulmonary resuscitation (CPR): An emergency procedure used to establish effective circulation and respiration to a victim whose heart has stopped beating

Emergency: An event that calls for immediate action

Gait belt: A strong and sturdy belt usually made of canvas material that is used to move, lift, or support residents by placing it securely around their waist

Geriatric chair or Geri chair: Chair with wheels and a tray attached to it

Hazard: A source of potential danger

Incident: An unusual event or occurrence

Immobile: Unable to move

Impairment: Anything that hinders proper function

Protective device: A type of restraint that keeps the resident from harm

Oxygen: A colorless, odorless gas that is essential for breathing

Restraints: Equipment used to protect, support, or hold a person in a particular position

Resident's unit: The space for one resident in a long-term care facility

Transfer belt: Same as gait belt

Resident Safety

As a nursing assistant, you must always make sure the residents are safe. All of the staff must be concerned for the safety of the resident. You should realize many of the residents are frail or weak due to disease or old age.

Some residents will have **impairments** in vision, hearing, or balance among other disabilities. These, along with less physical strength, may increase the chance of accident or injury. Other residents may have some mental impairment or may be confused. Any of these conditions puts the resident at higher risk of injury or accident. The newly admitted resident, who may not be familiar with the surroundings, will be another high-risk person.

Potential Hazards

Some of the more common **hazards** found in many long-term care facilities are the following:

- Hazardous substances such as disinfectants, cleaning supplies, medications, etc., that residents may touch if cabinets and storage areas are left unlocked or are easily accessible

- Lack of proper lighting. Glare is especially hazardous to the elderly person

- Unsafe equipment

- Slippery floors

- Unlocked wheelchairs, geriatric chairs, shower chairs, or beds

- Errors such as giving the resident the wrong tray, treatment, or medication

- Improper restraints and safety devices

- Improperly placed or nonworking call light

- Unsafe or improperly performed procedures

- Improper use of smoking materials
- Cluttered hallways

Prevention of Accidents

Preventing accidents is the responsibility of everyone in the health care facility. Many accidents can be prevented by an alert staff. By being aware of the hazards, you can prevent many accidents. Some of the ways the staff can prevent injuries or accidents to itself and residents are the following:

- Respond to emergency calls immediately

- Follow care plan at all times

- Answer call lights as soon as possible

- Check for proper identification when performing procedures

- Many injuries occur in the bathroom, be alert when toileting residents

- Use wheel locks on beds, lifts, wheelchairs

- Use side rails as indicated on care plan

- Use safety devices, restraints when indicated on care plan

- Clean up spills immediately

- Be alert for sharp objects and remove if indicated

- Be aware that glaring light affects the vision of the resident

- Cluttered hallways pose a threat to the resident

- Unsafe electrical use, extension cords

- Report unsafe equipment

- Know procedures and do them properly
  - Ask questions if you are unsure of task
  - Do not perform tasks you have not been taught

- Get help when necessary

- Know fire safety policy of facility. Be alert to fire safety violations. Know smoking rules, oxygen safety, electrical equipment, unsafe wires, overuse of extension cords

- Recognize that some residents cannot stay very long in the sunlight due to medications or medical conditions. Follow care plan

- Maintain your own health
  - Staff should stay away from facility when ill. Be sure to call facility when illness prevents your ability to work

- Use proper precautions when working with contaminated items

Falls

Falls are a serious threat or hazard to the resident. They are a frequent cause of accidents in the long-term care facility. If a resident falls while you are walking with him, you should do the following:

- Gently ease the resident to the floor (Figure 7-1).

- Guide the resident to the floor grasping the transfer belt. Or support the resident under the arms

- Lean the resident onto your leg as you go down to floor with resident

- Prevent the resident's head from hitting floor

Always call for the nurse immediately. Stay with the resident. Do not attempt to move the resident until the nurse has checked him.

Incidents

Anytime an accident or injury occurs, an incident report must be filled out. An **incident** can be described as any event that is not part of the routine care or routine operation of the health care facility. An incident may involve the resident, the staff, or visitors.

Restraints and Safety Devices

Restraints are **protective devices** that limit a resident's freedom to move about. These safety devices are an infringement on the resident's rights and may be used only when ordered by the physician. Restraints must be used only when absolutely necessary and when other means to protect the resident have not been successful.

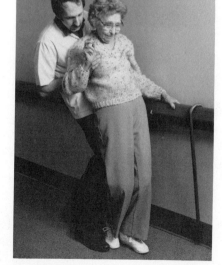

FIGURE 7-1.
If the resident falls, gently ease
her to the floor or ground.

Reasons for Using Restraints

Restraints are used for protecting the resident and should be used only when other methods to protect the resident have not been successful. Restraints may be applied:

- To prevent injury, such as falling

- To prevent the resident from injuring others

- To protect from pulling on tubing or wound coverings or some other safety measure

Types of Restraints

There are a variety of protective devices. Some of the more commonly used restraints in the long-term care facility are the following:

- side rails on beds

- vest or jacket (Figure 7-2)

- belts

- hand mitts

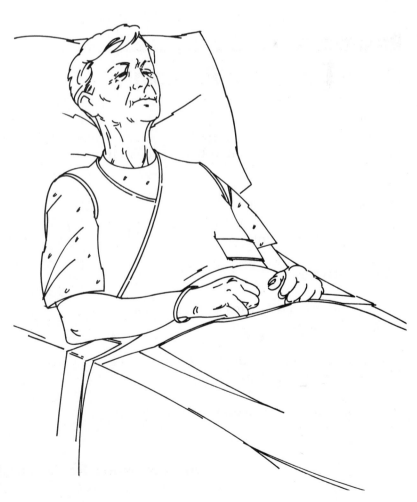

FIGURE 7-2.
Vest restraint with front closure.

- wrist

- geriatric chairs

Guidelines to observe when using restraints on residents are the following:

- The instruction must be written in the care plan with an order from the doctor

- The resident must be released every two hours at which time the resident must be allowed to walk or given range-of-motion exercises according to instructions on the care plan. This must be recorded on the resident's medical records

- Restraints must be used only if other means of protection or safety have not worked

- Apply the restraint properly. For example, vest restraints that tie in the front must not be used other ways

- Apply the restraint securely but do not cut off or restrict circulation

- Check for skin irritation

- Always explain to the resident the reason for restraint

Procedure 4

Applying a Vest Restraint

1. Wash your hands.

2. Explain to resident who you are and what you are going to do.

3. Get help, if necessary.

4. Get a vest restraint.

5. Give privacy.

6. Slip the resident's arms through the armholes of the vest.

7. Make sure clothing under restraint is not wrinkled and vest fits smoothly.

8. Fasten ties or secure vest to fit comfortably but not tightly.

9. Bring the straps through the slots at sides of vest.

10. Tie the straps of the vest to the bed frame or in the back of chair or wheelchair.

11. Use knot recommended by facility policy.

12. Place call light within resident's reach.

13. Leave resident comfortable and safe.

14. Wash your hands.

15. According to policy, record or report the resident's skin condition and reaction to restraint application.

(See Procedure Review, page 209)

Fire Safety

Your facility will have special fire safety procedures. All staff must watch for fire hazards and report them immediately to the proper authority. Because fire safety is extremely important, most states have laws requiring long-term care facilities to have frequent fire drills. Some of the major causes of fire in the long-term care facility are the following:

- Improper use of smoking materials

- Defects in heating systems

- Improper trash disposal

- Misuse of electrical equipment

- Spontaneous combustion

You should always be aware that in order for a fire to occur, three things must be present:

- Material that burns

- Flame or spark

- **Oxygen** in the air

Fire safety is very important when oxygen is being used. A tiny spark or a cigarette ash can cause a fire when oxygen is present in larger amounts than is normally present in the air. Special procedures must be followed when oxygen is used. Your facility will show you these procedures.

Actions to Take When You Discover Fire

- Follow the facility's procedures

- Follow facility policy for getting out **immobile** residents. This may include placing the resident on a blanket on the floor, and pulling the resident from danger or moving the entire bed with the resident in it

Many facilities use the "R A C E" system to serve as a general guideline in fire safety.

- Remove residents in immediate danger

- Alert other staff members

- Confine the fire

- Extinguish fire, if possible

Fire Extinguishers

When you begin your job, you will be shown the fire plan and the location of fire extinguishers (Figure 7-3 a, b). You will also be shown how to use the fire-fighting equipment. Three types of fire extinguishers commonly used are the following:

- Water, used for ordinary combustible fires

- Chemical, used for flammable liquid fires and electrical equipment fires

- Foam, used for flammable liquid fires

Body Mechanics

Body mechanics refers to the proper use of the muscles to make the best use of your strength and to avoid fatigue and injury to yourself or others. Using proper body mechanics is one of the safest things you can do to prevent injury to the resident and to yourself.

Importance of proper body mechanics

Nursing assistants move, lift and turn residents often in their daily work. Using proper body mechanics can prevent injuries and lessen strain and fatigue. Proper body mechanics also involves the following:

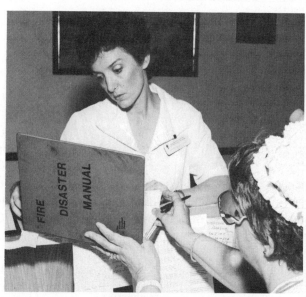

FIGURE 7-3a.
Know your facility's fire plan.

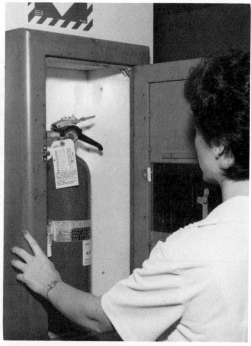

FIGURE 7-3b.
Know where the fire extinguishers are and how to use them.

- Using good posture and balance. The strongest muscles of the body do the work

- Using your own body and that of the resident

- Enhancing the safety, comfort, and confidence of the residents

Guidelines for Using Proper Body Mechanics

- Plan what you are going to do

- Explain the procedure to resident

- Get help, if necessary

- Have a wide base of support. Place your feet 12 to 14 inches apart

- Move close to the resident. Do not reach from a distance

- Use "internal girdle." Tighten your abdominal muscles upward and your buttocks muscles downward before lifting

- Squat to move or lift an object. Bend at knees and hips. Keep your back straight

- Lift by using thigh muscles

- Work smoothly and match your movements when working with a partner

- Turn with your feet. Do not twist your body

- Do not lift when you can push or pull

- Use lifting aids when appropriate, such as mechanical lifts and lift sheets.

Resident's Unit

When we speak of the **resident's unit**, we are referring to the area that is for a resident's personal use (Figure 7-4). The items in the unit are a bed, chair, table for over-bed use, bedside stand, dresser, closet, and sometimes a television set or radio. Many facilities allow some furniture items from the resident's former home if there is enough space. You must realize this is the resident's "home." Caring for the resident includes some caring for the unit.

The resident's personal items are very valuable because they bring back memories of the past. Handling these items with respect and care shows the resident you care. Showing respect for the resident's

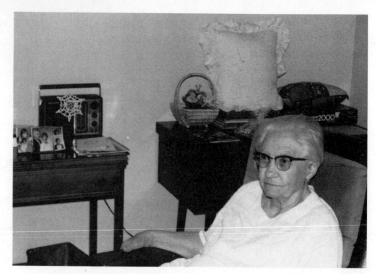

FIGURE 7-4.
The resident's unit is "home."
Treat it respectfully.

personal belongings is also one way you can help the resident with grief and loss issues.

The resident has a right to expect his or her unit be treated with respect and dignity. This includes knocking on closed doors and giving the resident and his visitors the right to privacy when requested.

Unit Safety

The nursing assistant must check the resident's unit each day for safety. Some considerations to note are as follows:

- Check side rails to be sure they are secure. These are used by resident to prevent falling when turning in bed

- Check call light. Make sure the light is working and within the resident's reach

- Keep unit tidy. Major cleaning is the job of other departments in most cases

- Always respect the resident's choices. Ask him how and where he wants items, if possible

- Respect resident's right to privacy when you clean closets and drawers

- Make the resident's bed (Figure 7-5)

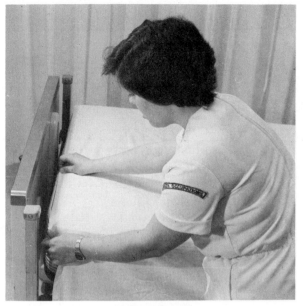

FIGURE 7-5a.
Position the small hem of the bottom sheet even
with the foot of the mattress.

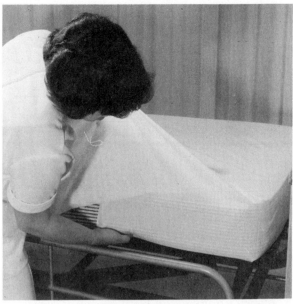

FIGURE 7-5b.
To make a mitered corner, pick up the sheet
about 12 inches from the head of the bed and
form a triangle with a 45-degree angle. Tuck the
lower portion under the mattress.

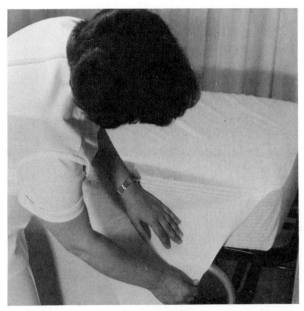

FIGURE 7-5c.
To finish the mitered corner, fold the triangle
down and tuck the final fold under the mattress.

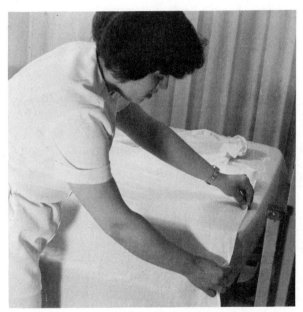

FIGURE 7-5d.
Position the top sheet on the bed with the wrong
side up and the wide hem even with the top edge
of the mattress.

Procedure 5

Making the Unoccupied Bed

1. Wash your hands.

2. Introduce yourself to the resident.

3. Explain to resident what you are going to do.

4. Gather supplies needed: two large sheets, linen draw sheet, plastic or rubber draw sheet, pillow case, laundry bag or hamper, and clean bedspread, if needed.

5. Carry linens away from your uniform.

6. Place linens on clean area near bed in order of use. From bottom to top: pillow case, spread, sheet, linen draw sheet, plastic draw sheet, and sheets).

7. Place bed in high, flat position.

8. Remove and fold spread if you are reusing it.

9. Remove soiled linens by rolling them into a ball without touching your uniform.

10. Place soiled linens in laundry bag.

11. Place bottom sheet on bed, centering the lengthwise middle fold of sheet in middle of bed.

12. Open sheet.

13. Place sheet with small hem even with foot edge of mattress.

14. Tuck top of sheet under top of mattress.

15. Miter corner of sheet at head of bed. Secure upper and lower corners of fitted sheet.

16. Tuck in bottom sheet on side of bed, working from head to foot.

17. Place plastic draw sheet over middle one third of bed.

18. Tuck edge of plastic sheet under mattress.

19. Place linen draw sheet over plastic sheet, covering entire plastic sheet.

20. Tuck linen draw sheet under mattress.

21. Place top sheet on bed, centering the lengthwise middle fold in center of bed.

22. Position sheet with top edge even with top of mattress.

23. Tuck bottom of sheet under mattress at foot of bed.

24. Place bedspread on bed.

25. Position bedspread about four inches above top edge of mattress.

26. Miter top linens at foot of bed.

27. Move to other side of bed.

28. Pull and smooth out bottom sheet.

29. Tuck bottom sheet under mattress at head of bed pulling tight.

30. Miter corner of sheet at head of bed. Secure upper and lower corners of fitted sheet.

31. Pull and tightly tuck side of bottom sheet under mattress.

32. Pull plastic sheet tightly.

33. Tuck plastic sheet under mattress, pulling and tucking from middle of plastic sheet first. Then pull and tuck edges of sheet.

34. Pull linen draw sheet tightly.

35. Tuck linen draw sheet under mattress, pulling and tucking from middle of draw sheet first. Then pull and tuck edges.

36. Check foundation of bed. Make sure bed is smooth and wrinkle free.

37. Pull and smooth top sheet.

38. Pull and smooth spread.

39. Tuck sheet and spread under foot of mattress.

40. Miter top linens at foot of bed.

41. Fold spread back about 30 inches.

42. Make cuff on top sheet by folding back about four inches at top edge of sheet.

43. Place pillow on bed.

44. Insert zippered end of pillow in pillowcase toward closed end of pillowcase.

45. Straighten pillowcase on pillow.

46. Place pillow at head of bed.

47. Cover pillow with bedspread.

48. Place bed in low position.

49. Place call light within resident's reach.

50. Assure resident's comfort and safety.

51. Wash your hands.

(See Procedure Review, page 211)

Emergency Measures

There may be times in the long-term care facility when emergency measures must be performed. Your facility will have a specific policy for emergency procedures. Your responsibility is to tell the nurse immediately and follow the nurse's instructions. Knowing some of the emergency procedures is important. You might want to consider taking a CPR/first aid course offered by a community organization.

Choking

○ If the resident is coughing and cannot speak and breathe, do not intervene

○ Establish that the resident's airway is obstructed
  • Clutching at his or her neck is the common, universal sign for choking
  • Ask the resident "are you choking?" If the resident nods yes, you must do something right away

Clearing an Obstructed Airway (Heimlich Maneuver)

Some of the residents in a long-term care facility cannot swallow very well. The best measure is to prevent choking, but even with the best care some residents may choke on food or other objects. The policy of facilities vary, but there are times when you may have to help the resident who is choking (Figure 7-6).

Procedure 6

Clearing an Obstructed Airway (Heimlich Maneuver)

Clearing an Obstructed Airway in a Conscious Adult:

1. Call for the nurse immediately.

2. If resident is sitting or standing, stand behind him.

3. Wrap your arms around his waist.

4. Make a fist with one hand.

5. Place the thumb of your fist against the resident's abdomen, just above the navel and below the tip of the breastbone.

6. Grasp fist with other hand.

7. Push in and upward on abdomen with a quick thrust.

8. Repeat until the foreign body comes out or resident loses consciousness. Proceed to CPR only if you've had instruction. Otherwise, call nurse.

Clearing an Obstructed Airway in an Unconscious Adult

It is extremely important that you know of your facility's policy regarding this procedure. Often this is the responsibility of the nurse. The procedure is listed here for your general understanding only.

1. Call for help, but do not leave.

2. Lower resident to the floor and position him on his back

3. Open airway by tilting head back and lifting jaw.

4. Use finger sweep to try to clear foreign object from mouth. Do not push it further down throat.

5. Try to give two breaths.

6. Straddle victim.

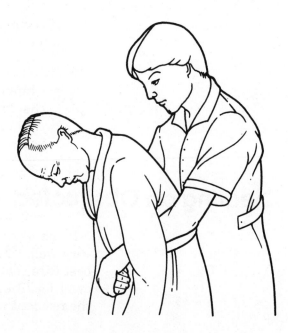

FIGURE 7-6.
Placement of hands for the
Heimlich maneuver.

7. Place heel of hand above navel. Thrust 6 to 10 times.

8. Try to give two breaths.

9. Repeat thrusts, sweeping mouth, and giving breaths until object is dislodged.

10. Continue until airway is open, help arrives, or rescuer cannot continue.

(See Procedure Review, page 215)

Cardiopulmonary Resuscitation (CPR) _____

Cardiopulmonary resuscitation (CPR) is a basic, lifesaving procedure given to a person whose heart suddenly stops. This is called cardiac or respiratory arrest. The techniques of CPR must be taught by a certified instructor. The following outline gives only an idea of the CPR procedures. It does not replace a CPR course.

- Shake resident and shout, "Are you all right"

- Turn victim on back

- Open airway. Look, listen, and feel for breath

- Use mouth-to-mouth breathing. Give two full breaths

- Feel for carotid pulse

- Begin chest compression, if there is no pulse

- Kneel beside resident's shoulders

- Position hands on chest correctly
  - Place heel of right hand over lower portion of breastbone, not on tip of breastbone or over ribs
  - Place left hand over right hand
  - Keep elbows straight

- Compress breastbone downward

- Continue compressions at rate of 60 per minute. If only one person is doing CPR, do15 compressions to 2 breaths per minute

Key Points in This Chapter

- Safety is very important in the long-term care facility, because many residents are at high risk for accidents or injuries.

- Accident prevention is the responsibility of the entire staff.

- Falls are a frequent cause of injury to residents.

- Incident reports must be made out whenever an accident occurs to a resident, staff member, or visitor.

- Restraints may be used only when other means of protection have not been successful.

- Restraints require a doctor's order and must be released every two hours.

- Fire safety is so important that most states require frequent fire drills for long-term care facilities.

- Body mechanics refer to proper use of your stronger muscles when moving or lifting.

- The unit is the resident's "home" and must be treated with respect.

- In an emergency situation, you must follow the instructions of the facility's policy.

Review Quiz Chapter 7
Comfort, Safety, and Emergency Measures

Choose the best answer for the questions below.

1. Which of the following may place the resident at high risk of injury?

   Ⓐ The alert resident
   Ⓑ The newly admitted resident
   Ⓒ The resident with vision impairment
   Ⓓ all of the above
   Ⓔ B and C only

2. Which is the safest way to prevent residents from having contact with hazardous substances, such as cleaning supplies and medications?

   Ⓐ Label containers with poison signs
   Ⓑ Tell the resident to stay away from hazardous materials
   Ⓒ Lock cabinets where hazardous materials are stored
   Ⓓ Tell other residents to watch any confused residents

3. Which of the following floor conditions pose a threat to resident safety?

   Ⓐ Colored carpeting
   Ⓑ Spilled liquids
   Ⓒ Tile floor
   Ⓓ Carpet

4. If the resident begins to fall while you are walking with him or her, you should

   Ⓐ leave the resident to get help.
   Ⓑ ask another resident to help you.
   Ⓒ gently ease the resident to the floor.
   Ⓓ get a pillow for the resident immediately.

5. What must be done when an event that does not fit the normal routine happens?

   Ⓐ An incident report must be made.
   Ⓑ The administrator of the facility must be notified.
   Ⓒ The resident must be restrained.
   Ⓓ An announcement must be made over the loudspeaker.

6. Which is true regarding the use of restraints?

   Ⓐ Restraints may be applied when the nursing staff is busy.
   Ⓑ Restraints may be applied only to residents who are confused.
   Ⓒ Restraints may be applied only if necessary to protect the resident from harm to himself or others.
   Ⓓ Restraints may be applied to all residents at night to keep them in bed.

7. How often should restraints be released?

   Ⓐ Once every shift
   Ⓑ Whenever requested by the resident
   Ⓒ Every four hours
   Ⓓ Every two hours

8. In order for a fire to occur, what must be present?

   Ⓐ Spark, oxygen, and material
   Ⓑ Flame and oxygen
   Ⓒ Oxygen and material
   Ⓓ Material and spark

9. In case of a fire, what should be done first?

   Ⓐ Call the fire department.
   Ⓑ Alert other staff.
   Ⓒ Remove residents in danger.
   Ⓓ Announce the fire over the loudspeaker.

10. Using good body mechanics does all of the following *except*

   Ⓐ prevents fatigue in the nursing assistant.

   Ⓑ reduces injury to the nursing assistant.

   Ⓒ reduces the risk of injury to the resident.

   Ⓓ increases the resident's strength.

11. Proper body mechanics includes

   Ⓐ having a wide base of support.

   Ⓑ using the back muscles to lift.

   Ⓒ keeping feet close together when lifting.

   Ⓓ keeping object to be lifted at arms' length from body.

12. The nursing assistant's responsibility for daily care of the unit includes

   Ⓐ washing the bed.

   Ⓑ mopping the floor.

   Ⓒ cleaning all bathroom equipment.

   Ⓓ checking for safety and proper working side rails and call lights.

13. When an emergency occurs in the long-term care facility, your responsibility as a nursing assistant is to

   Ⓐ notify the family immediately.

   Ⓑ follow directions of your supervisor.

   Ⓒ call the proper police or fire department.

   Ⓓ notify the administrator and follow their directions.

14. The universal sign for choking is

   Ⓐ clutching the neck.

   Ⓑ waving arms about.

   Ⓒ coughing.

   Ⓓ shouting.

15. If resident is coughing and able to breathe

   Ⓐ wrap your arms around resident's waist.

   Ⓑ stay with resident and let him continue coughing.

   Ⓒ use finger sweep to remove object causing coughing.

   Ⓓ give resident oxygen.

16. The correct procedure for clearing an obstructed airway in an unconscious adult is to place the heel of your hand

   Ⓐ on the chest.

   Ⓑ below navel.

   Ⓒ above navel.

   Ⓓ on the back.

17. One of the most frequent causes of accidents to residents in long-term care facilities is

   Ⓐ burns.

   Ⓑ falls.

   Ⓒ smoking.

   Ⓓ choking.

18. Accident prevention is the responsibility of the

   Ⓐ Maintenance Department.

   Ⓑ Administrator.

   Ⓒ Nursing Department.

   Ⓓ entire staff.

ANSWERS

1. E	6. C	11. A
2. C	7. D	12. D
3. B	8. A	13. B
4. C	9. C	14. A
5. A	10. D	15. B
		16. C
		17. B
		18. D

Chapter 8

Body Alignment and Activity Needs

In this chapter you will learn the importance of proper positioning, moving, and lifting of the resident. After reading this chapter you should be able to:

- Define Key Terms
- Describe Principles of Rehabilitation
- List Effects of Immobility
- Define Body Alignment
- List Guidelines to Follow when Moving or Lifting Residents
- Move and Position the Resident
- Ambulate the Resident Using a Cane and Walker
- Transfer the Resident
- Help the Resident Do Range-of-Motion Exercises

Key Terms

ADL: Activities of daily living, that include dressing, grooming, eating and moving about

Alignment: Proper body position as in good posture

Ambulate: To walk

Atrophy: Wasting away of muscle

Body mechanics: Proper use of the body to attain the most strength and reduce injury

Contracture: Abnormal tightening or shortening of muscles from lack of exercise

Edema: Swelling in the tissues often seen in legs, ankles, feet, and hands

Extend: To straighten out the joint

Flex: To bend the joint

Fowler's position: Sitting with head of bed elevated and knees bent

Hemiplegia: One half (right or left side) of the body is paralyzed

Immobility: Unable to move

Lateral position: Lying on side

Paralysis: Loss of ability to move a part or all of the body

Prone position: Lying on one's abdomen (stomach)

Prosthesis: Artificial body part

Range-of-motion (ROM) exercises: Exercises that move each muscle and joint

Rehabilitation: A process designed to restore and maintain a person's highest level of ability

Semi-Fowler's position: Similar to Fowler's position with head and knees slightly lower than in the Fowler's position

Side-lying position: Lying on one's side; lateral position

Supine position: Lying on one's back

Transfer: Moving from one surface to another, as in moving a resident from bed to wheelchair

Rehabilitation

Rehabilitation is the process designed to help a resident restore and maintain the highest level of physical and mental ability. As a nursing assistant, you will have a major role in the resident's rehabilitation program. The care plan will tell you your responsibility. Other members of the rehabilitation team will include the physical therapist, the occupational therapist, the speech therapist, and the activities department. Any program of rehabilitation will be based on the resident's physical condition and the resident's ability and desire to cooperate.

Three basic principles in rehabilitation programs are the following:

- Preventing more disability

- Keeping present strengths

- Restoring abilities lost by disease, illness, disuse, or the aging process

Some points to remember in any rehabilitation program include the following:

- Encourage self-help with **ADLs** by using adaptive equipment, such as a shoe horn or grippers

- Emphasize resident's abilities

- Encourage the resident in active **range-of-motion exercises** (moving limbs freely)

- Encourage resident to be as independent as possible if consistent with care plan

- Follow care plan for resident using **prosthesis** such as artificial leg or arm

Immobility Effects

Immobility affects the resident's physical and psychosocial needs. Try to understand how frustrated residents must feel when they always need help to move. Some residents will not be able to move at all without your help. Besides the mental frustrations, there are medical effects of inactivity on the body.

Physical Effects of Immobility:

Some of the physical problems seen in all body systems as a result of inactivity are the following:

○ **Circulatory System**
- Blood in vessels may tend to pool, causing blood clots
- Poor blood flow may cause **edema** (swelling) in tissues
- Increased work load for the heart

○ **Respiratory System**
- More difficult for lungs to expand
- Risk of lung infections is increased

○ **Urinary System**
- Without gravity urine tends to be retained in the bladder, causing urinary tract infection

○ **Digestive System**
- Loss of appetite
- Constipation

○ **Musculoskeletal System**
- Calcium loss is increased when stress is not placed on bones
- **Contractures** (shortening and tightening) of muscles occur in muscles that are not used
- **Atrophy** (wasting away of muscle tissue) results in weakness of muscle

○ **Integumentary (skin) System**
- Bedsores that reach deeper tissues develop easily on the resident who does not have frequent position changes

Mental and Social Effects of Immobility

Inactivity leads to loss of self-esteem, poor body image, and increased dependence on others. Inactivity is often a factor leading to depression. Most residents feel better if they have some interaction with others. The resident who cannot move about should be helped out of his room and should be around activity. Even the resident who is unable to see or hear will benefit from being around activity. Inactivity and immobility can lead to withdrawal, isolation, and loneliness. Instructions to help the immobile resident are found on the care plan.

Body Mechanics

You learned the importance of proper **body mechanics** in an earlier chapter. Since the topics covered in this chapter require lifting, transferring, and moving residents, body mechanics is again emphasized (Figure 8-1).

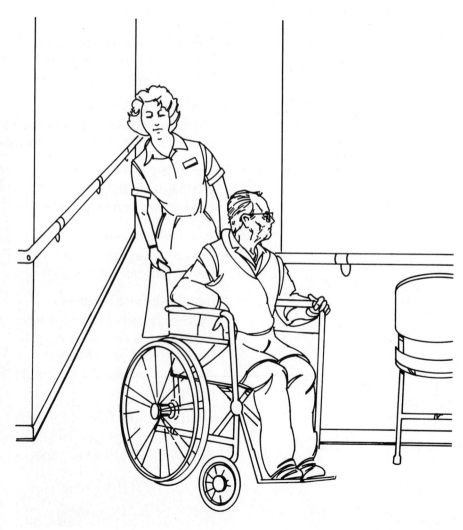

FIGURE 8-1.
Keep safety in mind when
moving a resident.

Importance of Proper Body Mechanics

Nursing assistants move, lift, and turn residents often in their daily work. Using proper body mechanics can prevent injuries and minimize strain and fatigue.

Proper body mechanics involves the following:

- Using good posture and balance. The strongest muscles of the body do the work

- Using your own body and that of the resident

- Enhances the resident's safety, comfort, and confidence

Guidelines for Using Proper Body Mechanics

- Plan what you are going to do

- Explain the procedure to resident

- Get help if necessary

- Have a wide base of support. Place your feet 12 to 14 inches apart (Figure 8-2)

FIGURE 8-2a. ▶
Keep your back straight and feet apart.

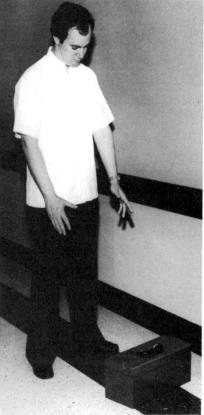

FIGURE 8-2b. ▼
Bend from the hips and knees when picking up an object.

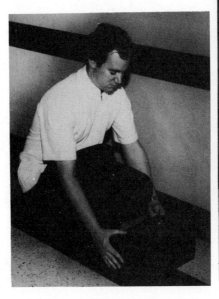

- Move close to the resident. Do not reach from a distance

- Use "internal girdle." Tighten you abdominal muscles upward and your buttocks muscles downward before lifting

- Squat to move or lift an object. Bend at knees and hips. Keep your back straight

- Lift by using thigh muscles

- Work smoothly and match your movements when working with a partner

- Turn with your feet. Do not twist your body

- Do not lift when you can push or pull

- Use lifting aids when appropriate, such as transfer belts, mechanical lifts, and lift sheets

Body Alignment

The correct positioning of the resident's body is referred to as **body alignment** (Figure 8-3). The resident should be positioned in good posture whether in a sitting or lying position. Always follow instructions from the supervising nurse or the resident's care plan. The following points refer to proper body alignment for positioning of the resident.

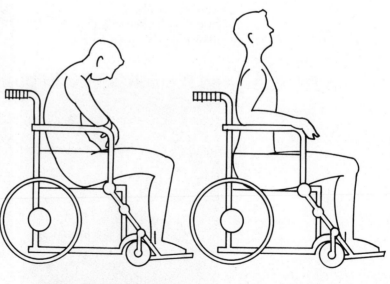

POOR ALIGNMENT   GOOD ALIGNMENT

FIGURE 8-3.
Body alignment.

Sitting in Bed (Fowler's position)

- Have the resident lie on his back with the head of bed and knees elevated

- Make sure resident's hips are at bend of bed

- If necessary, move resident up in bed at intervals

- If necessary, support arms with pillows

Sitting in a Chair

- Place resident's feet flat on floor or stool

- Position hips and knees at right angles

- Rest buttocks firmly against back of chair

- Position spine straight against back of chair

- Position resident's head directly over shoulders

- Support elbows on armrests

- If necessary, prop resident with pillows to maintain good alignment

Lying in Supine Position (lying on back)

- Place a small pillow under the resident's head. It usually allows for better alignment than a large pillow

- Keep the feet in proper alignment and prevent footdrop with a footboard

- Use positioning devices (handrolls, splints, foam or firm wedges), if indicated on care plan

Lying in Side-Lying Position or Lateral position

- Support upper arm and leg with pillows (Figure 8-4)

- Position upper leg so weight does not rest on lower leg

- Place a pillow lengthwise to support the resident's back and maintain the position

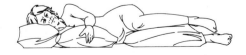

FIGURE 8-4.
Use pillows to provide support to the
upper arm and leg.

Lying in Prone Position (lying on abdomen)

Use this position for residents only if directed to do so by nurse or care plan.

- Turn the resident's head to one side when lying prone

- **Flex** resident's arms and position near resident's head

- Place the resident's feet in space between mattress and foot of bed

Procedure 7 _____

Positioning the Resident in Supine Position

1. Wash your hands.

2. Explain to resident who you are and what you are going to do.

3. Give privacy.

4. Lock bed wheels.

5. Raise bed to comfortable working level.

6. Lower side rail on working side after positioning bed.

7. Position resident, lying on his back.

8. Place resident's arms at sides in comfortable, functional position, supporting with pillows, if necessary.

9. Check for good body alignment.

10. Pad bony prominences of elbows and heels, if indicated.

11. Leave resident comfortable.

12. Raise side rails.

13. Position call light within resident's reach.

14. Place bed in low position.

15. Wash your hands.

16. Report to nurse or record any skin irritation or redness.

(See Procedure Review, page 217)

Procedure 8

Positioning a Resident in a Side-Lying Position

1. Wash your hands.

2. Explain to resident who you are and what you are going to do.

3. Gather supplies.

4. Give privacy.

5. Lock bed wheels.

6. Raise bed to comfortable working level.

7. Lower side rail on working side after positioning bed.

8. Begin this procedure by standing on the side opposite from which the resident will lie.

9. Use proper body mechanics to move resident.

10. Place one of your arms under resident's shoulder. Place other arm under resident's back.

11. Move upper part of resident's body towards you.

12. Place one of your arms under resident's waist and other arm under resident's thighs.

13. Move resident's midsection toward you.

14. Move resident's legs toward you.

15. Raise side rail.

16. Go to other side of bed. Lower side rail.

17. Flex and place resident's arm nearest you and toward head of bed. Place resident's other arm across chest.

18. Cross resident's leg farthest from you across nearest leg.

19. Place one of your hands on resident's shoulder. Place the other hand on hip.

20. Roll resident toward you.

21. Adjust pillow under resident's head.

22. Flex and place upper arm on pillow.

23. Place hand in functional position.

24. Flex and place upper leg on pillow. Upper leg and pillow should not rest on lower leg.

25. Raise side rail. Go to other side of bed.

26. Lower side rail.

27. Position pillow alongside resident's back.

28. Raise side rail.

29. Check for good alignment.

30. Pad bony prominences of elbows and heels, if indicated.

31. Leave resident comfortable.

32. Raise side rails.

33. Position call light within resident's reach.

34. Place bed in low position.

35. Wash your hands.

36. Report to nurse or record any skin irritation or redness.

(See Procedure Review, page 219)

Procedure 9

Moving a Resident Up in Bed

1. Wash your hands.

2. Introduce yourself to resident.

3. Explain to resident what you are going to do. Use good body mechanics throughout this procedure.

4. Provide privacy.

5. Lock bed wheels.

6. Raise bed to comfortable working level.

7. Lower head of bed.

8. Remove pillow from under resident's head.

9. Lean pillow against headboard.

10. Stand next to bed.

11. Ask resident to bend knees and put feet flat on mattress.

12. If resident is able, ask him to bend arms at sides. Place hands on bed. Push with hands when told to do so.

13. Slide one hand and arm under resident's upper back and shoulders.

14. Slide other arm under resident's hips and buttocks.

15. Instruct resident to push with hands and feet on count of three.

16. On count of three, move resident to head of bed.

17. Replace pillow under head.

18. Check to see if resident is in good alignment.

19. Raise side rail and lower bed.

20. Leave resident comfortable and safe with call light within reach.

21. Tidy area.

22. Wash your hands.

23. Record or report resident's tolerance to procedure and skin condition.

(See Procedure Review, page 221)

Transferring and Ambulating the Resident

You will be transferring, or moving, residents out of bed into wheelchairs several times a day. It is important that you do this correctly to avoid injury to the resident and to yourself. It is always good to practice these skills with another trainee or nursing assistant. Practice will reinforce and help you learn the rules of safety. Another task you will be expected to perform is to **ambulate**, or walk with, the resident. Using a transfer belt or gait belt helps assure the resident's and your safety.

A transfer belt is a heavy, canvas belt placed closely around the resident's waist. You can hold onto it while lifting the resident instead of lifting the resident under the arms. While ambulating the resident, a firm grasp on the transfer belt helps you ease the resident to the floor in case of a fall.

Guidelines for Moving and Lifting Residents

o Plan your moves
- Refer to care plan
- Explain procedure to resident making certain resident understands what is to be done
- Use a transfer belt to prevent injury to yourself and the resident
- Use lifting devices, if indicated
- Have bed at proper height
- Get assistance, if you are not sure the resident can safely move, position, or transfer

o Be alert to safety
- Use brakes on beds, wheelchairs, and lifts (Figure 8-5)
- Always make sure lifting or moving devices are in proper working condition
- When transferring a resident, move resident toward his stronger side
- Support resident's weaker side when transferring
- Be alert to catheter tubing safety
- Make sure surfaces are stable
- Have resident wear nonskid shoes, if possible
- Put on artificial limbs and braces properly
- Avoid lifting the resident under the arms. This can dislocate the resident's shoulders
- Support body parts when turning resident
- Approach corners slowly and watch for cross traffic
- Check canes and walkers for safety before using them
- Observe and report any changes such as:
  o dizziness, unsteadiness, inability
  o signs of skin irritation
  o resident's comments

o Psychosocial concerns
- Let the resident help as much as possible if consistent with care plan
- Encourage resident to be in charge of moving
- Ask resident to count to three
- Offer resident choices, such as where and when to be moved
- Realize that the inability to move is a great loss of the resident's independence
- Know the resident's fears, such as falling or being left alone

Procedure 10

Ambulating the Resident with a Walker or Cane

1. Wash your hands.

2. Explain to resident who you are and what you are going to do. Use good body mechanics throughout this procedure.

3. Gather supplies: cane or walker (Figure 8-6), transfer belt, resident's robe, and shoes, if necessary.

4. Give privacy.

5. Lock bed wheels.

6. Check cane or walker for safety.

7. If resident is in bed, lower side rail.

8. Raise head of bed.

9. Help resident sit on edge of bed by supporting shoulders while resident swings legs across and off side of bed.

10. Help resident into robe and shoes.

11. Put transfer belt around resident's waist, fitting closely and securely.

12. Put cane in resident's hand or walker in front of resident.

13. Help resident stand. Grasp the transfer belt underhand at resident's side.

14. When resident is standing and is balanced, ask him if he is dizzy or weak.

15. Walk beside resident. Hold transfer belt at resident's back.

16. Walk distance recommended by care plan or nurse's instruction.

17. Encourage resident to walk with back straight and head up.

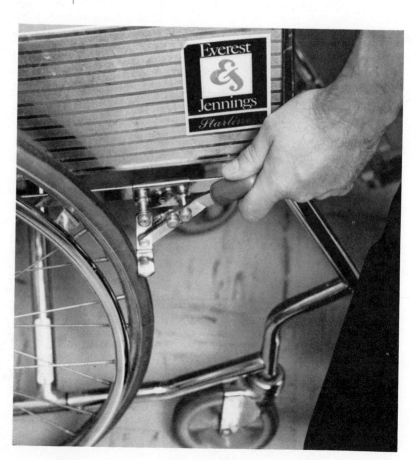

FIGURE 8-5.
Make sure wheelchair brakes work well.

18. Help the resident to a chair or bed.

19. Remove transfer belt. Remove robe and shoes, if resident is returning to bed.

20. Raise side rails, if resident is returned to bed.

21. Leave resident comfortable and safe with call light within reach.

22. Replace equipment, and tidy area.

23. Wash your hands.

24. Record or report distance walked and resident's tolerance.

(See Procedure Review, page 223)

Procedure 11

Transferring a Resident from Bed to Wheelchair

1. Wash your hands.

2. Explain to resident who you are and what you are going to do. Use good body mechanics throughout this procedure.

3. Gather supplies: wheelchair, transfer belt, resident's robe, shoes or slippers, and covering for lap.

4. Give privacy.

5. Position wheelchair so resident's stronger side will be closest to wheelchair when resident is sitting on edge of bed. Place wheelchair within one foot of bed at slight angle.

6. Raise or remove foot rests. Lock wheelchair brakes.

7. Raise head of bed.

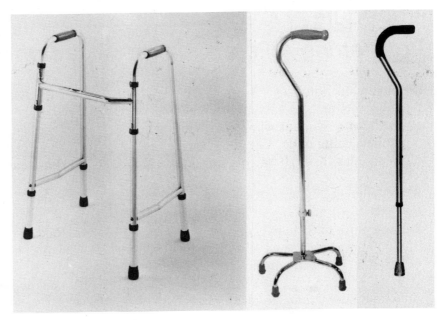

FIGURE 8-6.
Walkers and canes help residents to walk or "ambulate."

8. Lock bed brakes. Lower side rail.

9. Put on resident's shoes or slippers.

10. Cross weaker leg over stronger leg.

11. Help resident sit on edge of bed.

12. Check whether resident seems weak.

13. Help resident put on robe.

14. Put transfer belt securely around resident's waist.

15. Use transfer belt to move resident to edge of bed until resident's feet are flat on floor.

16. Grasp transfer belt at resident's waist with both hands, using an underhand grasp.

17. Support resident's weaker side.

18. Tell resident to push off bed with his stronger hand after counting to three.

19. Help resident stand.

20. Turn resident to wheelchair toward his stronger side. Keep a good grasp on transfer belt with both hands.

21. Be sure that resident can feel edge of wheelchair seat before he sits.

22. Tell resident to place stronger hand on wheelchair arm. Sit resident in chair.

23. Remove transfer belt.

24. Put wheelchair safety belt on the resident.

25. Adjust wheelchair leg rests and footrests.

26. Place resident's feet on footrests.

27. Cover lap with covering.

28. Leave resident comfortable and safe with call light within reach.

29. Replace equipment. Tidy area.

30. Wash your hands.

31. Record or report resident's tolerance and ability.

(See Procedure Review, page 225)

Procedure 12

Transferring a Resident from Wheelchair to Toilet

1. Wash your hands.

2. Explain to resident who you are and what you are going to do. Use good body mechanics throughout this procedure.

3. Give privacy.

4. Make sure bathroom is empty.

5. Bring resident in wheelchair to bathroom.

6. Close bathroom door.

7. Position wheelchair at right angle to toilet. That is, the side of the wheelchair faces the front of the toilet.

8. Release wheelchair security belt.

9. Fasten transfer belt around resident's waist, if required.

10. Lock wheelchair brakes.

11. Tell resident to push up from wheelchair while you lift him with transfer belt. Count to three to match movements.

12. Ask resident to hold bathroom grab bar.

13. Help resident stand, giving him time to get balanced.

14. Turn resident so he is standing in front of toilet.

15. Lower resident's underwear.

16. Help resident sit on toilet.

17. Be sure call light is close to resident.

18. Give privacy.

19. Return when resident says he is done.

20. Put on gloves to help the resident wipe excess bowel movement or urine.

21. To help him stand, ask resident to hold onto bathroom grab bar and pull himself up. Match movements on the count of three. Grasp onto transfer belt at resident's waist.

22. Pull underwear up.

23. Smooth the resident's clothing.

24. Turn and seat resident into locked wheelchair.

25. Help resident wash hands.

26. Remove resident from bathroom.

27. Take off transfer belt.

28. Take resident where he wants to go.

29. Place call light within resident's reach.

30. Leave resident comfortable and safe.

31. Tidy area.

32. Wash your hands.

33. Record or report resident's tolerance to procedure and any unusual urine or stool.

(See Procedure Review, page 227)

Range-of-Motion Exercises

There may be times when you must give range-of-motion exercises to a resident. **Range of motion** is how far a joint is capable of being moved. A person's range of motion is affected by many things: age, body size, genetics, and the absence or presence of disease. You will only help the resident do range-of-motion exercises when told to do so by the nurse or when indicated on the care plan. In some facilities this is not the task of the nursing assistant. Ask for help if you are not certain of how to do range-of-motion exercises.

Purpose of Range-of-Motion Exercises

Range-of-motion exercises are performed for residents who are unable to move their own joints. There are several reasons for these exercises. Muscles not being used **atrophy**, become weak, and develop **contractures**. Doing the exercises for the residents who cannot exercise themselves is called **Passive range-of-motion exercises**. Some of the reasons these exercises are performed are the following:

- To prevent deformities
- To prevent pain
- To maintain normal function
- To increase joint motion
- To increase circulation
- To promote a sense of well-being

Guidelines for Doing Range-of-Motion Exercises

- Follow care plan instructions
- Explain procedure to resident
- Use good body mechanics
- Expose only the body part being exercised
- Support the limbs above and below the joint being exercised
- Do not push the joint pass the point of pain or resistance
- Watch resident's face for indication of pain or discomfort
- Do each exercise 3 to 5 times
- Encourage the resident to help with exercises, if indicated on care plan

Procedure 13

Giving Passive Range-of-Motion Exercises

1. Explain to resident who you are and what you are going to do.

2. Use good body mechanics throughout this procedure.

3. Wash your hands.

4. Give privacy.

5. Raise bed to comfortable working height.

6. Lower side rail on working side.

7. Position resident in supine position.

8. Exercise the extremities as indicated on care plan, supporting the limbs at closest joints.

   A. Head and neck:

     1. Lean head forward, bringing chin to chest.

     2. Lean head backward with chin up.

     3. Turn head from side to side.

     4. Turn head back and forth in a circular motion.

   B. Shoulders, arms, and elbows (Figure 8-7):

     1. Move arm over head, with arm touching top of head.

2. Return arm to side.

3. Move arm across chest.

4. Return arm to side.

5. Move arm straight up.

6. Return arm to side.

7. Bring arm away from body at side to shoulder level

8. Return arm to side.

9. With arm straight out at the side, bend at elbow and rotate shoulder.

10. Return arm to side.

11. Bend at elbow and bring hand to chin.

12. Return arm to side.

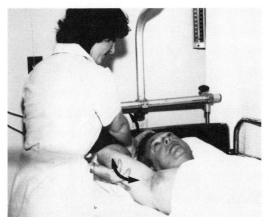 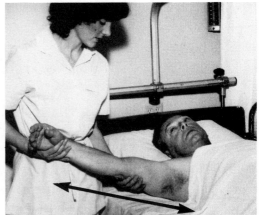

FIGURES 8-7a and 8-7b.
Range-of-motion exercises for the shoulder.

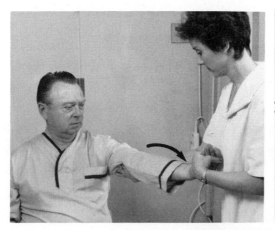 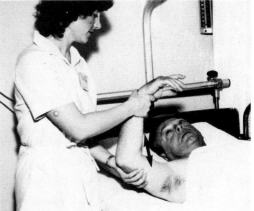

FIGURES 8-7c and 8-7d.
Range-of-motion exercises for the elbow.

C. Wrists, fingers, and forearms (Figure 8-8):

1. Bend hand backward at the wrist.

2. Bend hand forward at the wrist.

3. Clench fingers and thumb tightly as if making a fist.

4. Extend fingers and thumb.

5. Move fingers and thumb together and then apart.

6. **Flex** and **extend** joints in thumb and fingers.

7. Move each finger and thumb in a circular motion.

8. Extend arm along side of body with palm facing upward.

9. Rotate forearm with palm facing upward then downward.

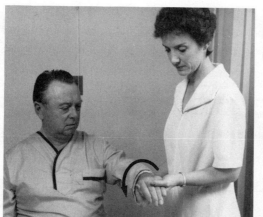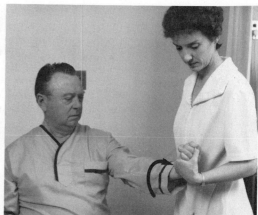

FIGURES 8-8a and 8-8b.
Range-of-motion exercises for the wrist.

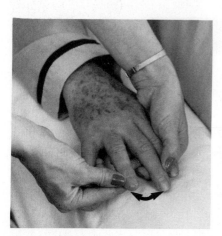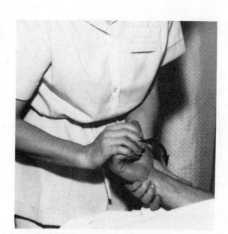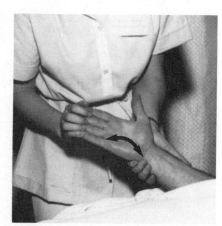

FIGURES 8-8c, 8-8d and 8-8e.
Range-of-motion exercises for the fingers.

D. Legs, hips, and knees (Figure 8-9):

1. Stretch leg out from the body.
   Return leg to other leg crossing
   over other leg only at ankle.

2. Bend and straighten knee.

FIGURES 8-9a-f.
Range-of-motion exercises for the hip and knee.

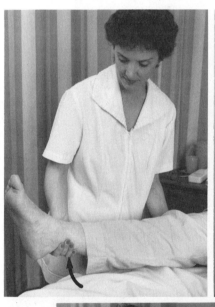 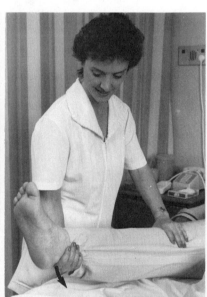 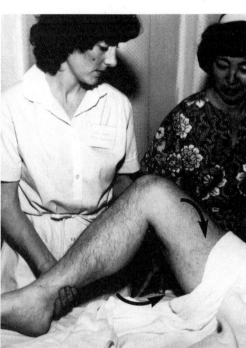

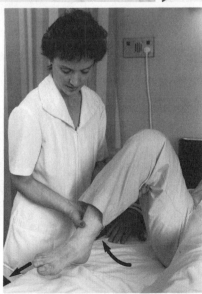 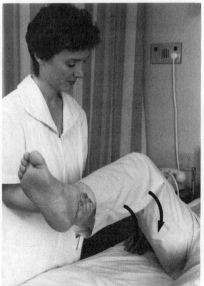 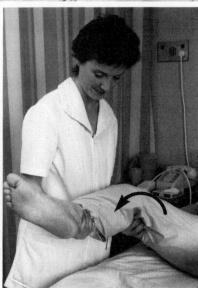

E. Ankles and toes (Figures 8-10 and 8-11):

    1. With leg straight on bed, push foot and toes toward front of leg.

    2. Push foot and toes out straight with toes straight. Point towards foot of bed.

    3. With leg straight, turn foot and ankle from side to side.

    4. Curl toes downward and upward.

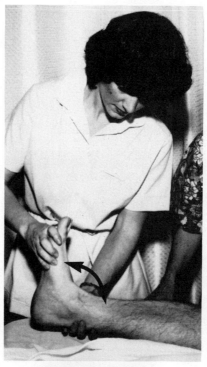

FIGURES 8-10a-b.
Range-of-motion exercises for the ankles.

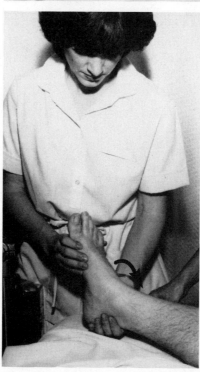
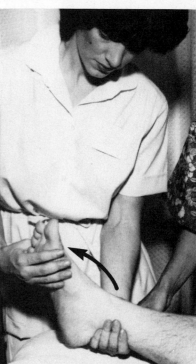

FIGURES 8-10c-d.
Range-of-motion exercises for the ankles.

9. Repeat each exercise as indicated on care plan.

10. Note resident's response to exercise.

11. Raise side rail. Lower bed.

12. Place call light within resident's reach.

13. Leave resident comfortable and safe.

14. Tidy area.

15. Wash your hands.

16. Record or report resident's tolerance to procedure.

(See Procedure Review, page 229)

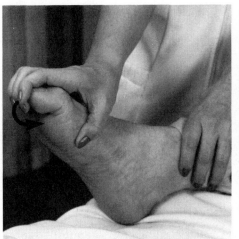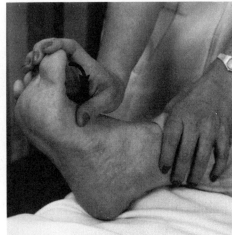

FIGURES 8-11a and 8-11b.
Range-of-motion exercises for the toes.

Key Points in This Chapter

- Rehabilitation is the process designed to restore and maintain the resident's highest level of ability.

- Immobility leads to break down of all body systems.

- Proper body alignment is necessary for the resident while sitting or lying down.

- Using a transfer belt helps prevent injury to the nursing assistant and the resident.

- Always follow the care plan when moving and lifting residents.

- Range-of-motion exercises are done to prevent physical problems in the resident with limited movement.

- Safety is important when moving or lifting residents.

Body Alignment and Activity Needs

Choose the best answer for the questions below.

1. The process designed to help a person restore and maintain his highest level of ability is

   Ⓐ range of motion.
   Ⓑ rehabilitation.
   Ⓒ restoration.
   Ⓓ assistance.

2. Maintenance, prevention, and restoration of abilities are the principles of

   Ⓐ adaptive devices.
   Ⓑ nursing care.
   Ⓒ rehabilitation.
   Ⓓ activity therapy.

3. What is a prosthesis?

   Ⓐ A mechanical lift
   Ⓑ A walker or cane
   Ⓒ An adaptive tool
   Ⓓ An artificial body part

4. All of the following statements are true *except*

   Ⓐ immobility affects the resident physically.
   Ⓑ there are mental effects from the resident's inability to move about.
   Ⓒ only the circulatory system is affected by immobility.
   Ⓓ residents may feel frustrated when they must rely on others to move about.

5. An effect of immobility on the circulatory system may be

   Ⓐ swelling in the tissues due to poor blood flow.
   Ⓑ constipation and loss of appetite.
   Ⓒ development of a bladder infection.
   Ⓓ loss of calcium in the bones.

6. Body alignment is

   Ⓐ lifting and moving residents.
   Ⓑ positioning the body in good posture.
   Ⓒ comfortable positioning for the nursing assistant.
   Ⓓ ways to use the muscles to the best ability.

7. What is the correct positioning for the resident when sitting in a chair?

   Ⓐ Feet should not be flat on floor.
   Ⓑ Hips should be at right angle in chair.
   Ⓒ Knees should always be straight out.
   Ⓓ Spine should be slanted into a half-lying position.

8. What does supine position mean?

   Ⓐ Lying on one's back
   Ⓑ Lying on one's side
   Ⓒ Lying on one's abdomen
   Ⓓ Lying on side with pillows supporting the spine

9. When a resident is in prone position, he or she is lying on the

   Ⓐ abdomen.
   Ⓑ side.
   Ⓒ back.
   Ⓓ back and side.

10. When moving a resident up in bed, ask the resident to help by

(A) pulling on side rails.
(B) pushing pillow up.
(C) straightening out legs and pushing with feet.
(D) bending knees, placing feet flat on bed, and pushing with feet.

11. When moving a resident up in bed, the pillow should be

(A) placed against the headboard.
(B) placed on a chair nearby.
(C) put out of way at the foot of the bed.
(D) kept under the resident's head when doing the moving.

12. A belt that is placed around the resident's waist when transferring him is called

(A) a lifting belt.
(B) a transfer or gait belt.
(C) a mechanical lifter.
(D) the moving or lifter belt.

13. Which of the following is *not* a true statement regarding lifting and moving residents?

(A) There is no need to explain procedures to a resident.
(B) Refer to care plan for special instructions.
(C) Make sure that equipment used for lifting or moving is working properly.
(D) Get help, if necessary.

14. When the resident has a weak side, it is best to move him or her

(A) with the weak side moving first to strengthen weaker side.
(B) with either side moving first.
(C) toward the weaker side.
(D) toward the stronger side.

15. Passive range-of-motion exercises are done for the resident

(A) who is up and about.
(B) who can move well without help.
(C) who cannot exercise himself.
(D) by another resident in the facility.

16. What must be your major concern(s) when moving or lifting a resident?

(A) How good the resident looks when finished
(B) How quickly you can do the task
(C) Safety of the resident
(D) All of the above

ANSWERS 1. B   2. C   3. D
4. C   5. A   6. B   7. B
8. A   9. A   10. D   11. A
12. B   13. A   14. D   15. C
16. C

111

Chapter 9
Personal Care Needs

In this chapter you will learn the importance of giving personal care to the residents. After reading of this chapter you should be able to:

- Define Key Terms
- Describe the Goals of Skin Care
- Identify Guidelines for Personal Care of the Resident
- Perform Oral Hygiene for the Resident
- Bathe the Resident
- Help Groom the Resident
- Measure Height and Weight
- Apply Support Hosiery
- Make an Occupied Bed

Key Terms

Abrasion: A rubbing away or scraping of the skin

Anti-embolism stockings: Elastic stockings that improve circulation by compressing the veins in the legs

Anus: The outlet for the rectum

Axilla: The armpit

Decubitus Ulcer: A pressure sore or bedsore

Decubiti: More than one bedsore

Dentures: Artificial teeth, may be partial or complete, upper or lower dentures

Genital area: The area which includes the external sex organs and the anus

Incontinent: Unable to control the discharge of urine or stool

Perineal (Peri-Care): Same as genital area

Pressure sore: Same as bedsore, decubitus ulcer

Prosthesis: An artificial body part

Skin Care

The skin is the largest organ of the body, and it performs several necessary functions (Figure 9-1). The skin is a protective outer covering that protects a person from infection and injury. The skin also removes water, salt, and waste through sweat. At certain places the skin joins with mucous membranes to line body openings. The hair and nails are considered part of the skin system.

As a nursing assistant you will give skin care to residents. It is important for you to know the changes caused by aging.

Age-Related Changes in the Skin

As in every body system, aging brings some changes in the skin, hair, and nails. The changes vary due to individual lifestyle, but generally the age-related changes in the skin are the following:

- The skin becomes drier, scaly, thin, and wrinkled

- The skin loses elasticity

- The fatty tissue under the layer of skin decreases

- Less oil and sweat are produced

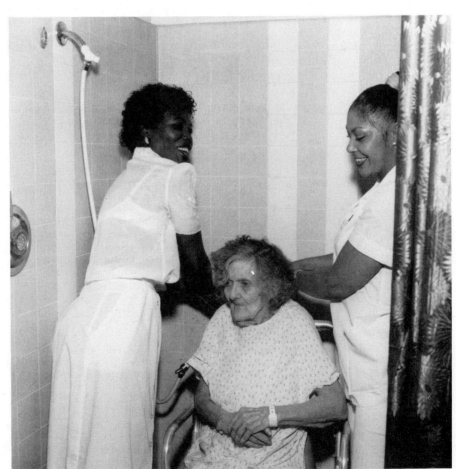

FIGURE 9-1.
Nursing assistants give residents a lot of the personal care.

- Skin tags and moles are more common

- The skin is less sensitive to heat, cold, and pain

- The skin becomes fragile, easily damaged, or torn

- The fingernails and toenails become thicker and brittle, and crack easily

Goals of Skin Care

The resident's care plan will state specific skin care goals, but some general goals are important for you to observe when giving skin care.

An elderly person's skin produces less oil, so the skin is often dry and flaky. For this reason, it is not necessary for most elderly people to have a bath every day. In fact, bathing every day often makes the skin drier. Most residents will have a partial bath at least once a day, but a full bath or shower is usually given only once or twice a week. The resident's care plan will tell you the bathing schedule.

When a person perspires, or sweats, the drops on the surface of the skin can pick up dirt and dust that mix with tiny flakes of skin. This warm, dark, and damp skin area give bacteria the chance to grow and spread. For this reason, cleaning the resident's skin is one of your major responsibilities. The major goals of bathing or cleaning the resident are the following:

- Cleanliness
  - Removing bacteria on skin
  - Removing sweat and other body secretions
  - Removing body odors

- Stimulate circulation
  - Warm water on the surface of skin increases blood flow
  - Light skin stroking helps blood flow
  - Massage soothes and stimulates the skin

- Mild exercise for resident
  - Moving body trunk, arms, and legs is mild exercise

- Observation—Thoroughly inspect the skin, report any signs of:
  - irritation
  - texture change
  - color change
  - growth
  - injury
  - pressure sores
  - drainage

- The chance to have personal, therapeutic communication with the resident

- Feeling of well-being
  - The feeling of being clean is refreshing and adds to the dignity and self-worth of the resident

Decubitus Ulcers

Bedsores are called **decubitus ulcers**, **pressure sores** or **decubiti**. They develop quickly in the immobile, elderly resident. Your observation and reporting skills must be acute in this area. Prevention is the best treatment of decubiti (Figure 9-2). Some important points regarding decubitus ulcers are the following:

- Pressure areas frequently develop over areas of bony prominences (Figure 9-3)
  - shoulder blades
  - spine
  - hips
  - tailbone
  - ankles
  - heels
  - elbows
  - ears
  - scalp

- Stages of decubiti
  - redness
  - pale or white skin
  - skin breakdown
  - blisters
  - deep tissue involvement

- Prevention
  - Keep resident up and walking about as long as possible
  - Change position at least every two hours
  - Massage skin over bony areas

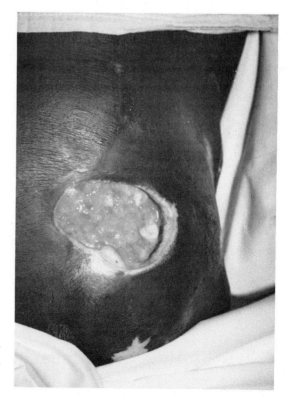

FIGURE 9-2.
Decubitus ulcer with deep tissue involvement.

- Keep skin clean and dry
- Help resident drink enough liquids and eat correctly
- Keep linens wrinkle free
- Follow nurse's or care plan instructions for special treatment of pressure sores
- Wear gloves

○ Observe and report immediately
  - redness of the skin
  - blisters
  - skin tears or **abrasions**
  - pain or tenderness
  - bruises
  - any skin color changes

○ Use pressure-relieving devices. Some examples of pressure-relieving devices are the following:
  - sheepskin
  - protective elbow and heel pads
  - bed cradles
  - alternating pressure mattress

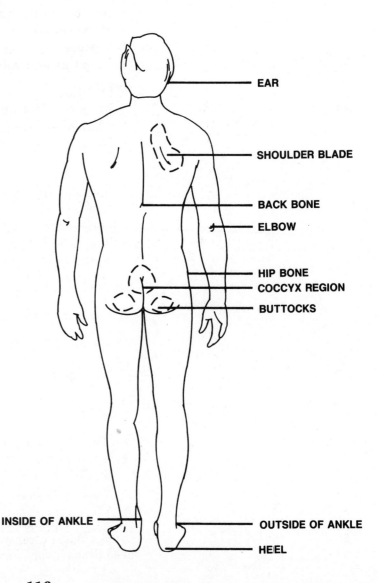

FIGURE 9-3.
Areas of pressure.

- egg crate foam mattress
- flotation mattress

Follow care plan when using these devices. Changing the resident's position often is necessary. Also, use any pressure-relieving device.

Personal Care _____

Personal care of the resident includes care of the mouth and teeth, hair, nails, and feet. It also is bathing, dressing, and grooming the resident. You will be responsible for helping the resident with these activities of daily living (ADL).

The resident has done his or her own personal care all his life. It may take longer to let the resident wash his own face and brush his own teeth, but you will add to the resident's self-worth by helping the resident, rather than doing it for him. Letting the resident be as independent as possible is one of the goals of good nursing care.

General Guidelines to Personal Care

○ Bathing should be a good cleaning of the body in a pleasant, relaxed area

○ Refer to care plan for special instructions

○ Give resident choices as often as possible. Schedule time for personal care according to the resident's needs and desires

○ Let resident to do as much as possible for himself, as indicated in care plan

○ Use adaptive devices that help resident to dress and groom himself. Adaptive devices include the following:
- long handle shoe horn
- long handled grippers
- adaptive brushes and combs

○ Protect resident's privacy

○ Dress resident in appropriate clothing

○ Avoid cold or exposure

○ Avoid overuse of powders or talc

○ Dry very well with special attention to skin folds and body creases

○ Be alert to safety concerns
- Transfer resident using transfer belt
- Test bath's water temperature
- Use safety belts on tub lifts
- Make certain bath mats are secure
- Help resident in and out of tub or shower
- Stay with resident in tub or shower

○ Wear gloves, if indicated

○ Report anything unusual to the nurse

○ Record procedure as indicated by facility policy

Oral Hygiene

Oral hygiene is the cleaning of the mouth, teeth, gums, and tongue. The purpose of oral hygiene is to remove food particles and reduce the number of bacteria in the mouth. One of your responsibilities is to provide good mouth care and cleanliness for the resident. A clean mouth helps prevent mouth odor and tooth decay. A feeling of well-being is created when a person has good oral hygiene.

Another purpose of providing oral hygiene is observation. While brushing the resident's teeth, you have an opportunity to observe the mouth (Figure 9-4). Some points to remember when giving oral hygiene are the following:

○ Encourage self-care if consistent with care plan

○ Let resident brush own teeth. Get supplies ready and take resident into bathroom in wheelchair

○ Wear gloves when doing oral hygiene

○ Clean comatose resident's mouth
  • Always explain procedure to resident even if resident appears unresponsive
  • Turn resident's head to side when cleaning the mouth of the unconscious to avoid getting liquids into lungs

○ Observe and report any signs of irritation, sores, lose teeth, or pain

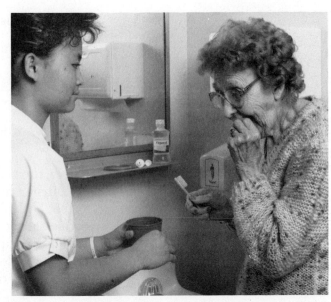

FIGURE 9-4.
Help the resident with dental care.

Denture Care

Many of the residents in a long-term care facility have **dentures** (false teeth). Dentures may be the entire set of teeth or only a few teeth. Dentures are necessary for eating, retaining the shape of the face and jaw and for giving the resident a sense of well-being.

Losing teeth can be depressing to some people. Many residents will try to keep others from seeing them without their dentures in place. Always respect the resident's privacy when giving denture care. Be very careful when handling dentures. Dentures are very expensive and can break if dropped. Some points to remember regarding denture care are the following:

- Wear gloves

- Remove dentures carefully. Let the resident remove them, if possible

- Brush dentures very well. Hold them securely

- Check dentures for cracks, chips, or loose teeth

- Let resident rinse or clean mouth before replacing dentures

- Store dentures in marked denture cup

- Always respect the resident's privacy

Procedure 14

Brushing the Resident's Teeth

1. Wash your hands.

2. Explain to resident who you are and what you are going to do.

3. Gather supplies needed: toothbrush, toothpaste, water, mouthwash, emesis basin, towel, and disposable gloves.

4. Place equipment on over-bed table.

5. Give privacy.

6. Raise bed to comfortable working height.

7. Elevate head of bed.

8. Lower side rail.

9. Put on gloves.

10. Place towel across resident's chest.

11. Help resident in self-care, if possible.

12. Moisten toothbrush. Apply toothpaste.

13. Brush resident's teeth using circular motion to all surfaces. Brush gums, tongue, sides, and roof of mouth.

14. Let resident rinse mouth with water or mouthwash.

15. Hold emesis basin while resident spits.

16. Wipe mouth with towel.

17. Check mouth for sores, redness, or irritation.

18. Raise side rail.

19. Lower bed.

20. Leave resident comfortable.

21. Place call light within resident's reach.

22. Clean and replace equipment.

23. Wash your hands.

24. Report or record the condition of mouth.

(See Procedure Review, page 233)

Bathing the Resident

The resident in a long-term care facility usually needs help bathing. Most residents have a full bath only once or twice a week, but most residents receive a partial bath at least once a day. The care plan will tell you what type of bath to give the resident and when to give the bath.

Types of Baths

Residents who are able will get a tub or shower bath. Most long-term care facilities have a bathroom that has a lift-over tub, which cleans as well as tub or shower bathing. A special shower chair is used for residents getting showers. A shampoo is often given at the same time as the bath. Refer to care plan if resident is to have hair washed while having bath.

Residents either too weak or ill to receive a tub or shower are given a bed bath. A nursing assistant cleans the resident's entire body, one part at a time while the resident remains in bed.

A partial bath is usually given to residents at least daily. A partial bath includes washing of face, hands, underarms, back, and genital area. The procedures for giving a bed bath and partial bath with perineal care follow later in this chapter.

Perineal Care

Perineal care also called **Peri-Care** refers to the washing and drying thoroughly of the **genital area**. In the female the genital area is the urinary opening, the vagina, and the rectum. In the male, the penis, scrotum, and rectum are included. For the resident who is **incontinent** peri-care must be given frequently. Urine or stool on the skin causes the already frail skin of the elderly person to break down quicker. Some points relating to peri-care are the following

- Wear gloves

- Realize many older people are very modest or embarrassed about having others clean their genital area

- Give care that protects the resident's modesty by giving privacy and exposing only the body part you are cleaning. Be sure privacy curtain is closed when giving this very personal care

- Wash properly, using warm soapy water. Rinse and dry thoroughly Some nursing homes may use special products for peri-care. Follow the facility's policy

- Wash catheter gently to remove urine, stool, or mucous

- You will be expected to give perineal care to both male and female residents in most cases

Procedure 15
Giving a Bed Bath

1. Wash your hands.

2. Explain to resident who you are and what you are going to do.

3. Gather supplies needed: basin, soap, washcloth, two towels, clean gown, bath blanket, lotion, comb or brush, and gloves.

4. Place supplies on clean area near bed.

5. Check room temperature of room. Make sure resident is not cold.

6. Give privacy.

7. Offer bedpan or urinal to resident.

8. Raise bed to comfortable working height.

9. Lower side rail.

10. Remove bedspread and blanket. Fold them and place on chair.

11. Place bath blanket over top sheet. Remove sheet without exposing resident. Place soiled sheet in hamper or on chair in room.

12. Remove resident's gown.

13. Raise side rail.

14. Fill basin with warm water.

15. Return to bedside. Lower side rail.

16. Place towel under chin.

17. Offer washcloth to resident to wash own face, if possible.

18. Make a mitten by folding washcloth around your hand.

19. Wash resident's eyelids from inner side of eye to outer side of eye.

20. Rinse cloth.

21. Wash face, neck, and ears.

22. Dry washed areas.

23. Place towel under resident's arm farthest from you.

24. Hold resident's arm up. Wash the whole arm from wrist to shoulder.

25. Rinse and dry arm.

26. Wash, rinse, and dry **axilla** (armpit).

27. Repeat for other arm.

28. If possible, place resident's hands in water. Wash, rinse, and dry hands, fingers, and nails.

29. Place towel across chest. Pull bath blanket down to abdomen.

30. Move towel to expose chest.

31. Wash, rinse, and dry chest.

32. Cover chest with towel.

33. Expose abdomen.

34. Wash, rinse, and dry abdomen.

35. Return bath blanket to resident's shoulders.

36. Remove towel from under blanket.

37. Uncover leg farthest from you. Place towel under leg.

38. Wash, rinse, and dry leg.

39. Repeat for other leg.

40. If possible, place feet in basin one at a time.

41. Wash, rinse, and dry feet.

42. Cover legs with bath blanket.

43. Raise side rail.

44. Empty basin and refill with clean water.

45. Lower side rail.

46. Ask resident to turn back toward you. Help him, if necessary.

47. Wash, rinse, and dry back.

48. Put lotion on back, massaging body prominences of hips, tailbone, spine, and shoulders.

49. Use gloves to wash genital area. Wash from front of genital area to rectal area.

50. Help resident into clean gown.

51. Comb hair. Help with other grooming requests.

52. Replace bed linens, if indicated.

53. Position resident comfortably. Put call light within resident's reach.

54. Raise side rail. Lower bed.

55. Clean and replace equipment.

56. Dispose of soiled linens.

57. Wash your hands.

58. Report or record skin condition and resident's tolerance.

(See Procedure Review, page 235)

Procedure 16

Giving a Partial Bath With Perineal Care

1. Wash your hands.

2. Explain to resident who you are and what you are going to do.

3. Gather supplies needed: basin, soap, washcloth, two towels, bath blanket, clean gown or clothing, comb or brush, and gloves.

4. Place supplies on clean area near bed.

5. Check room temperature. Make sure resident is not cold.

6. Give privacy.

7. Offer bedpan or urinal to resident.

8. Raise bed to comfortable working height.

9. Lower side rail.

10. Remove bedspread and blanket. Fold them and place on chair or fold at foot of bed.

11. Place bath blanket over top sheet. Remove sheet without exposing resident. Place soiled sheet in hamper or on chair. Fold clean sheet to foot of bed.

12. Raise side rail.

13. Fill basin with warm water.

14. Return to bedside. Lower side rail.

15. Remove resident's gown.

16. Place towel under chin.

17. Offer washcloth to resident to wash own face, if possible.

18. Make a mitten by folding washcloth around your hand.

19. Wash resident's eyelids from inner side to outer side of eye.

20. Rinse cloth.

21. Wash face, neck, and ears.

22. Dry washed areas.

23. Place towel under hand farthest from you.

24. If possible place resident's hand in basin. Wash, rinse, and dry hand.

25. Repeat for other hand.

26. Wash, rinse, and dry axilla (armpit).

27. Repeat for other armpit.

28. Help resident to turn his back to you.

29. Wash, rinse, and dry upper back.

30. Wash, rinse, and dry buttocks.

31. Put lotion on back, massaging bony prominences of hips, tailbone, spine, and shoulders.

32. Put on gloves.

33. Wash perineal area.

   o Female
   - Lift leg closer to you. Place on pillow, if necessary
   - Wash genital area from front to back, separating labia.
   - Wash area around **anus** last.
   - Rinse and dry very well.

   o Male
   - Help him to lie on his back.
   - Wash penis, pubic area, and scrotum.
   - If he is not circumcised, gently draw foreskin back and clean head of penis. Replace foreskin.
   - Rinse and dry very well.
   - Position male on his side to clean anus and anal area.

34. Cover resident.

35. Dress resident appropriately.

36. Help grooming requests.

37. Position resident comfortably. Put call light within resident's reach.

38. Raise side rail. Lower bed.

39. Clean and replace equipment.

40. Throw out soiled linens.

41. Wash your hands.

42. Report or record resident's skin condition and tolerance.

(See Procedure Review, page 239)

Applying Lotion to the Resident

Another part of good skin care is massaging the skin with lotion. Always refer to the care plan. If indicated, massage the resident's skin with light, smooth strokes. Massage can stimulate circulation and is often recommended over the bony prominences.

Procedure 17

Applying Lotion to the Resident

1. Wash your hands.

2. Explain to resident who you are and what you are going to do.

3. Gather supplies: lotion and towel.

4. Provide privacy.

5. Raise bed to working height.

6. Lower side rail.

7. Help resident turn on side, facing away from you.

8. Expose back.

9. Place towel along side of back.

10. Pour small amount of lotion into hand, warm lotion with hand.

11. Apply lotion to back. Pay special attention to bony prominences along spine, shoulders, hips, and tailbone.

12. Continue to massage with smooth strokes until lotion is rubbed into skin.

13. Wipe off extra lotion.

14. Smooth and straighten bottom linens.

15. Cover resident, and position him comfortably.

16. If indicated, apply lotion to other pressure areas of skin, such as elbows and feet.

17. Leave resident comfortable and safe.

18. Place call light within resident's reach.

19. Raise side rail.

20. Lower bed.

21. Tidy area. Throw away linens.

22. Wash your hands.

23. Record or report redness or skin irritation.

(See Procedure Review, page 243)

Grooming The Resident

Grooming the resident includes combing hair, shaving, nail care, and putting glasses or hearing aids in place (Figure 9-5). Self-esteem is increased when one is well groomed. Some points to remember when grooming the resident are the following:

- Give choices, if possible
- Encourage self-care, if possible
- Give privacy
- Dress and groom resident appropriately
- Clean items after using them: shaver, comb, brush
- Help resident clean eye-glasses. Handle the glasses with care
- Care for the resident's hearing aid, if necessary
  - Follow manufacturer's or the care plan instructions for cleaning and inserting hearing aid

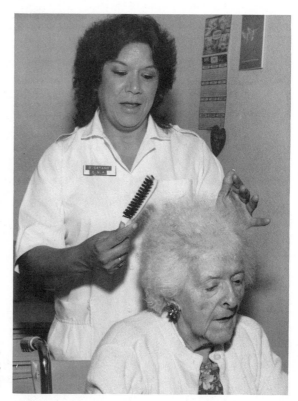

FIGURE 9-5.
Hair care is an important part of daily grooming.

- Make sure batteries are working. A whistling sound should be heard when volume is checked
- Insert hearing aid properly
- Clean hearing aid properly, and handle it with care. Usually warm soapy water is used to wash the outside parts of hearing aids

Prosthesis Care

A **prosthesis** is an artificial body part. Prosthetic devices such as artificial legs, arms, or breast can make life much more enjoyable for the person using it. You will find some residents in the long-term care facility who wear a prosthesis. Some points to remember when caring for the resident who wears a prosthesis are the following:

- Refer to care plan for special instructions

- Remember this is part of the resident's body and needs to be cared for as such

- Wash prosthesis

- Be alert to pressure areas under prosthesis. Check for redness, irritation, and blisters

- Dress resident wearing prosthesis properly. Stockinette is usually worn under artificial limbs

- Report to nurse if you notice that prosthesis needs repair

- An artificial eye is usually cared for by nurse. If you are instructed to care for the resident with an artificial eye, handle it very carefully. The artificial eye socket and the eye must be cleaned as indicated on care plan

Foot Care

Special care is sometimes part of caring for the resident's feet. Because poor blood circulation to the feet is common, the skin on the resident's feet heals slowly if injured. Injury prevention is often the best treatment in caring for the feet. Some points to follow regarding foot care are the following:

- Follow care plan instructions

- Trim nails more easily after soaking them

- Soak feet often. Dry very well, and put on lotion often

- Cut resident's toenails only when told to do so by nurse. Some residents may need a podiatrist, a foot doctor

- Do not cut the diabetic resident's toenails. This is usually not the nursing assistant's responsibility

Applying Support Hosiery

Support hosiery is for the resident who has circulation problems. The hose provide some pressure on the legs, which helps increase the blood flow. These stockings are made of stretchable elastic and fit very closely. Support stockings may be knee length or cover the entire leg. These types of hosiery are called **anti-embolism stockings** or often referred to by the brand name TED Sox. Some points to remember about support hosiery or anti-embolism stockings are the following:

- Follow care plan as to when stockings are to be put on and for how long resident is to wear the hosiery

- Put stockings on resident before he or she gets out of bed in the morning

- Must be applied smoothly with no wrinkles

- Make sure hosiery is the correct size

- Hosiery must fit very well to be effective

Procedure 18

Applying Support Hosiery

1. Wash your hands.

2. Explain to resident who you are and what you are going to do.

3. Gather stockings of proper size.

4. Give privacy.

5. Help resident lie down.

6. Expose one leg at a time.

7. Grasp stocking with both hands at the top opening and roll or gather toward toe end.

8. Adjust stocking over toes, foot, and heel.

9. Apply stocking to leg by rolling or pulling upward over the leg.

10. Make sure stocking is on evenly. Be sure there are no wrinkles.

11. Expose other leg.

12. Grasp stocking with both hands at the top opening and roll or gather toward toe end.

13. Adjust stocking over toes, foot, and heel.

14. Apply stocking to leg by rolling or pulling upward over the leg.

15. Make sure stocking is on evenly. Be sure there are no wrinkles.

16. Leave resident comfortable and safe.

17. Place call light within resident's reach.

18. Wash your hands.

19. Report or record procedure.

(See Procedure Review, page 245)

Measuring and Recording Height and Weight _____

Measuring the resident's height and weight is one of the nursing assistant's responsibilities in the long-term care facility. Some of the points to remember when doing this procedure are the following:

- ○ Refer to the resident's care plan or follow nurse's instructions regarding method and time

- ○ Methods of weighing residents
  - Standing scale. Resident must be able to stand without help
  - Chair scale. The scale is manufactured with a chair permanently mounted on it
  - Wheelchair scale. You must weigh wheelchair without resident before weighing him in wheelchair. The weight of chair is subtracted

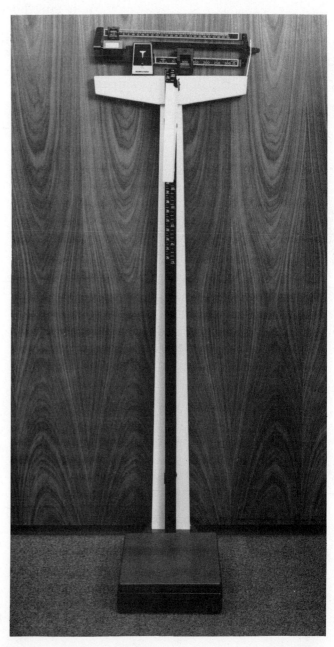

FIGURE 9-6.
Scale must be level to
be accurate.

- Electronic scales
- Bed scale is used for residents who cannot get out of bed

○ Methods of measuring height
  - Standing scale usually has height indicator and can be used for the resident who can stand
  - Tape measure is used for residents who cannot stand

○ Guidelines for weight and height measurements (Figure 9-6)
  - Weigh residents at the same time of day
  - Use the same scale each time the resident is weighed
  - Be certain scales are balanced before weighing
  - Have resident wearing similar clothing each time they are weighed

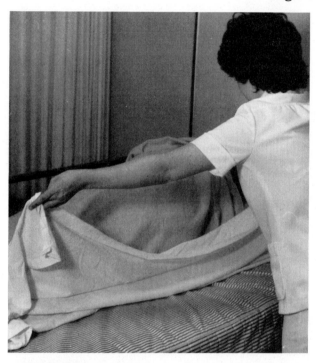
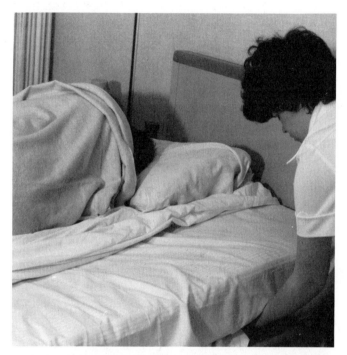

FIGURES 9-7a-b. ▲
After fanfolding the clean top sheet at the center of the bed, make a mitered corner and tuck the sheet in place from the head to the foot of the bed.

FIGURE 9-7c. ▶
Make a toepleat (room for the toes) in the top linen by folding a three-inch section of the linen towards the foot of the bed.

- Follow policy of facility when recording height and weight of resident

Making the Occupied Bed

There may be times when you will have to change the sheets and make the entire bed while the resident is in it (Figure 9-7). This is done for residents restricted to bed rest. That is, those who are too weak or ill to get out of bed. Other times you will change only some of the linens while the resident remains in bed.

Procedure 19

Making the Occupied Bed

1. Wash your hands.

2. Explain to resident who you are and what you are going to do.

3. Gather supplies needed: two large sheets, linen draw sheet, plastic or rubber draw sheet, bath blanket, pillow case, laundry bag or hamper, clean bedspread, and blanket, if needed.

4. Hold linens away from your uniform.

5. Place supplies on clean area near bed in order of use. From top to bottom: pillow case, spread, sheet, linen draw sheet, plastic or rubber draw sheet, and sheets.

6. Provide privacy for resident.

7. Raise bed to comfortable working height. Lock wheels of bed.

8. Lower side rail on working side. Make sure other side rail is secure.

9. Remove bedspread and blanket. Fold and place on chair.

10. Place bath blanket over top sheet. Remove sheet without exposing resident. Place soiled sheet in hamper or on chair in room. Or, if not using bath blanket, leave top sheet covering resident.

11. Help resident to turn on side away from you.

12. Loosen bottom linens.

13. Roll soiled draw sheet and rubber sheet and tuck along resident's back.

14. Roll soiled bottom sheet and tuck along resident's back under the draw sheet and rubber sheet.

15. Place clean sheet on bed with center fold at center of bed.

16. Unfold one half of sheet.

17. Place bottom hem of sheet even with edge of mattress. Or, fit corner of fitted sheet.

18. Tuck top of sheet under half of head end of mattress.

19. Miter corner of top sheet. Or, fit corner of fitted sheet.

20. Tuck sheet under side of entire mattress, working from head to foot of bed.

21. Roll remaining half of sheet and tuck under soiled sheet.

22. Place rubber draw sheet in the middle of bed. Tuck in at side of bed.

23. Place clean linen draw sheet over rubber draw sheet. Tuck in at side of bed.

24. Roll remaining halves of draw sheets and tuck along resident's back under the soiled sheets.

25. Help resident roll over linen pile to side facing you.

26. Raise side rail.

27. Go to other side of bed.

28. Lower side rail.

29. Loosen and remove soiled linens from under mattress.

30. Place soiled linens on chair or in hamper. *Do not put linens on floor.*

31. Pull clean bottom sheet over mattress.

32. Tuck the bottom sheet tight under head of mattress.

33. Miter corner of sheet at head of bed. Or, fit corner of fitted sheet.

34. Pull bottom sheet tight, and tuck under side of mattress, working from head to foot of bed.

35. Pull rubber sheet tight, and tuck over bottom sheet at side of mattress.

36. Pull draw sheet tight, and tuck over rubber sheet at side of mattress.

37. Help the resident to roll on back. Place bath blanket or bed sheet on resident.

38. Place clean sheet over bath blanket or bed sheet, centering center fold of sheet.

39. Pull bath blanket or soiled sheet from under clean sheet.

40. Place blanket and bedspread over sheet.

41. Fold top sheet over edge of blanket. Spread to make a cuff with sheet.

42. Tuck top linens under foot of mattress, giving "toe room" for resident's feet.

43. Miter the corner of top linens at foot of bed.

44. Raise side rail.

45. Go to other side of bed.

46. Tuck top linens under mattress at foot of bed.

47. Miter corner of top linens at foot of bed, giving "toe room" for resident's feet.

48. Remove pillow and soiled pillowcase.

49. Place clean pillowcase on pillow.

50. Replace pillow under resident's head.

51. Leave resident comfortable and safe.

52. Place call light within resident's reach.

53. Raise side rail.

54. Lower bed.

55. Tidy area. Put linens in hamper.

56. Wash your hands.

57. Record or report resident's tolerance to procedure.

(See Procedure Review, page 247)

Key Points in This Chapter

- The skin in the elderly is more fragile, tears and breaks readily, and is more easily damaged.

- The skin in the elderly produces less oil, which causes dry, sometimes flaky skin.

- Decubitus ulcers are breaks in skin caused from pressure.

- Changing the resident's position is the best prevention of decubitus ulcers.

- Encourage residents to do as much of their personal care as possible, if consistent with care plan.

- An important responsibility of the nursing assistant is observing and reporting any redness or other signs of skin irritation.

- The resident's self-esteem can be increased by appropriate clothing and attractive grooming.

- Anti-embolism stockings, which must be applied when the resident is lying down, must fit very well and smoothly to be effective.

Review Quiz Chapter 9
Personal Care Needs

Choose the best answer for the questions below.

1. Which is the largest organ in the body and provides it with a protective covering?

   (A) Skin
   (B) Hair
   (C) Nails
   (D) Heart

2. Age-related changes in the skin include

   (A) drier skin.
   (B) thicker nails.
   (C) more oil.
   (D) All of the above
   (E) A and B only

3. All of the following are goals of skin care *except*

   (A) removal of bacteria on skin.
   (B) removal of perspiration and other body discharges.
   (C) to stimulate blood circulation.
   (D) exercise for the nursing assistant.

4. Another term for bedsores is

   (A) mucous membranes.
   (B) decubiti.
   (C) cyanosis.
   (D) sores.

5. Which of the following help prevent bedsores?

   (A) Changing the resident's position often
   (B) Keeping linens wrinkle free
   (C) Giving adequate intake of fluids
   (D) All of the above

6. A sign of a pressure sore developing is

   (A) area of redness on skin.
   (B) foul smelling breath.
   (C) change in bowel habits.
   (D) pain in the chest.

7. What is included in oral hygiene?

   (A) A complete bedbath and linen change
   (B) Cleaning of the mouth, teeth, and gums
   (C) Helping the resident walk or be ambulatory
   (D) Cleaning and disinfecting the resident's bathroom

8. Which of the following is true about dentures?

   (A) Dentures should be cleaned while in the resident's mouth.
   (B) Dentures should be removed when eating.
   (C) Dentures are expensive and can break if dropped.
   (D) Only the nurse should handle the resident's dentures.

9. You are assigned to care for Mrs. White. She cannot walk, spends most of her day in the wheelchair, and is able to use her hands and arms well. What is the best way for you to help her brush her teeth?

   (A) Brush her teeth for her while she is in bed.
   (B) Brush her teeth for her after she is up in wheelchair.
   (C) Get the nurse to help her brush her teeth.
   (D) Help her brush her own teeth by taking her to the bathroom and getting the supplies she needs.

10. Which of the following should be done when giving a partial bath to Mrs. White?

   Ⓐ Take her to the shower to give a partial bath.
   Ⓑ Let her do as much of her care as possible, if consistent with care plan.
   Ⓒ Also help her comb her hair and put on makeup after giving partial bath.
   Ⓓ All of the above
   Ⓔ B and C only

11. What is perineal care?

   Ⓐ Cleaning the genital area
   Ⓑ Combing the hair of the resident
   Ⓒ Cleaning the tub and bathroom
   Ⓓ Cleaning the fingernails and toenails

12. Before inserting a hearing aid

   Ⓐ wash the hearing aid in alcohol.
   Ⓑ soak the hearing aid in cold water.
   Ⓒ make sure the batteries are working.
   Ⓓ ask the family how to operate the hearing aid.

13. Anti-embolism stockings should be put on the resident

   Ⓐ after the resident has been walking about.
   Ⓑ so the stockings fit loosely.
   Ⓒ when the resident is lying down.
   Ⓓ only at night.

14. Which of the following scales will need to be used for the resident who cannot stand without assistance?

   Ⓐ A chair scale
   Ⓑ A scale over the bed
   Ⓒ A standing scale
   Ⓓ Any of the above

15. When is an occupied bed made?

   Ⓐ Whenever the resident is in the room
   Ⓑ When the resident is on bed-rest restriction
   Ⓒ When all the linens must be changed
   Ⓓ When the resident has a complete bath

Chapter 10

Nutrition and Fluid Needs

In this chapter you will learn the importance of your role in helping the resident with good nutrition. After reading this chapter you should be able to:

- Define Key Terms
- Describe Proper Nutrition
- Identify Factors Affecting the Nutrition of the Resident
- Describe Special Diets
- Describe Importance of Fluid Balance
- Feed a Resident
- Identify Alternative Means of Meeting Nutritional Needs of Residents
- Record Intake and Output

Key Terms

Aspiration: The breathing of liquid or food into the air passages.

Cubic centimeter (cc): A metric unit of measurement; 30 cc. equal 1 ounce.

Dehydration: A condition in which the body has less than the normal amount of fluid.

Digestion: The process by which food is broken down in the body and changed into usable forms.

Edema: Abnormal swelling in the tissues caused by fluid retention.

Emesis: Vomiting or what is vomited.

Intake and Output: The recording of the amount of fluid taken and the amount of fluid lost by a person.

Intravenous: Within a vein

Milliliter (ml): A metric unit of measurement; 30 ml equal 1 ounce

Nutrients: Chemical substances necessary for life found in food.

Ounce: A unit of measurement equal to 30 cc. or 30 ml.

Therapeutic diet: A special or modified diet used to treat a person's individual situation.

Proper Nutrition

Proper nutrition is important for everyone. An adequate intake of proper foods and fluids is necessary to live and grow in a healthy manner. The **nutrients** in foods provide the necessary elements we need for growth and energy. There are six nutrients essential to good nutrition:

- proteins
- carbohydrates
- fats
- water
- vitamins
- minerals

Proper nutrition is enough intake of these nutrients. The four basic food groups serve as a guide to proper nutrition.

Food Groups

A balanced diet contains the essential nutrients. Eating the right number of servings from each food group is a balanced diet. Included below is a listing of the food groups, number of servings per day and why these nutrients are necessary.

- Meat, Fish, and Poultry
  - Two servings per day
  - Needed for growth, and to build and repair body tissues

- Milk Products
  - Two servings per day
  - Needed for healthy bones and teeth

- Cereals, Breads and Grains
  - Four servings per day
  - Needed for energy, cell development and to fight infection

- Vegetables and Fruits
  - Four servings per day
  - Needed for energy, and healthy tissues, bones and teeth

Water

Water is so necessary to life that a person can live only a few days without water. Adequate intake of fluids is required to replace fluids that are lost through urine, stool, sweat, and skin evaporation. The normal adult intake of fluids should be 2 to 3 quarts a day.

Offering liquids to the resident frequently is extremely important for the following reasons:

- Many residents are not able to drink liquids without your help

- Sense of thirst is less in elderly

- Adequate fluid intake is necessary to prevent urinary problems and constipation

Vitamins and Minerals

A person must have enough vitamins and minerals to stay healthy. Therefore, a regular diet should provide the necessary vitamins and minerals in a healthy adult.

What Affects the Resident's Nutrition

Nutritional needs of the older person are the same as the younger adult. However, meeting these needs can be more difficult for the elderly person (Figure 10-1). Often the resident in the long-term care facility depends on your help in receiving proper nutrition. Some factors to consider that affect the nutrition of the elderly resident are the following:

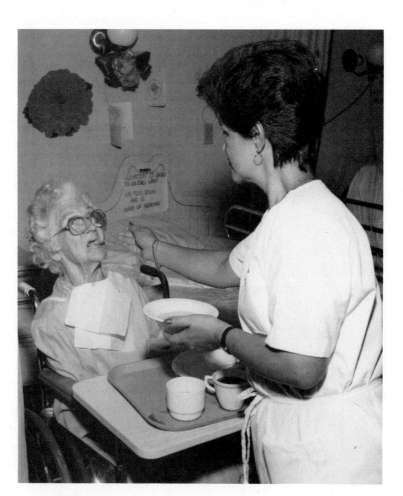

FIGURE 10-1.
Some residents will
need help eating.

- General health
  - Fatigue level
  - Level of alertness
  - Absence or presence of disease

- Sensory loss
  - Decreased taste, smell, and vision. Meals may need to be enhanced with proper seasonings unless against diet regulations listed on the resident's care plan
  - Sight, smell, taste and even the sound of food preparation affect appetite

- Physical comfort
  - Assure resident's comfort
  - Position properly to prevent **aspiration** or choking on foods

- Dentures
  - Improperly fitting dentures impair the resident's ability to enjoy mealtime
  - Be sure resident has dentures in properly at mealtime

- Ability to chew and swallow
  - Residents who cannot chew or swallow require special diets or procedures such as puréed foods or even tube feeding
  - Residents who cannot swallow easily have a very hard time with eating

- Cultural influences may affect the resident's nutrition. Some common cultural influences that affect the food choices of the resident are the following:
  - Religion
  - National cultures
  - Family customs
  - Economic backgrounds

- Emotional concerns affect the resident's eating habits. Common emotional states that affect eating habits are the following:
  - Loneliness
  - Depression
  - Anger, frustration

- Eating environment affects nutrition
  - Mealtime can be a source of social contact
  - All staff members can make mealtime pleasant
  - Pleasant table mates and conversation at mealtime are important
  - Too much noise in the dining room can be a problem. Avoid shouting and clanging dishes

Special Diets

Most of the residents will be on a general or regular diet. The dietitian in the long-term care facility plans meals for the residents. The dietitian makes menu changes for residents on special diets. Knowledge of special diets and **therapeutic diets** will help you understand their importance. Common therapeutic diets in the long-term care facility are the following:

- ○ Clear liquids
  - • Used for persons who have stomach or intestinal distress or as first foods after surgery
  - • Clear liquids include tea, broth, gelatin (Jello), some fruit juices and some soda pops
  - • Not generally used for residents with swallowing problems

- ○ Full liquid
  - • Given to residents who have digestive disorders
  - • Full liquid is clear liquids plus milk, custards, cream soups, ice cream and sherbet

- ○ Purée or Mechanical Soft
  - • Used for persons who cannot chew well
  - • Same as regular diet but food has been ground or chopped finely

- ○ Diabetic diet or calorie controlled—Ordered for the person who has diabetes or who is on a calorie-restricted diet
  - • No sugar on tray
  - • No foods with high sugar content
    - ○ honey
    - ○ syrup
    - ○ regular soda pops
    - ○ jelly, jams
    - ○ candy
  - • May have special sugar-free substitutes, if indicated on diet plan

- ○ Low Sodium (low salt)
  - • Used for persons with high blood pressure, heart, or kidney disease
  - • No salt on tray
  - • Limits foods high in salt such as
    - ○ bacon
    - ○ ham
    - ○ luncheon meats
    - ○ some cheeses and soups
    - ○ many common snacks

Fluid Balance

Proper fluid balance occurs when the loss of body fluids is about the same as the amount of fluid taken in. The nursing assistant has an important role in helping the resident maintain proper fluid balance. Some of the reasons for proper fluid balance are the following:

- ○ Helps proper blood flow

- ○ Helps food digestion

- Improves proper removal of body waste
- Protects cells by keeping
  - skin moist
  - mouth and throat moist
  - eyeballs moist
- Regulates body temperature
- Water makes up more than one half of body weight

Dehydration

Dehydration occurs when there is not enough fluid in the body. This condition may cause serious harm to vital body organs. Death will occur when there is severe body fluid loss. Some of the signs of dehydration are the following:

- Mouth becomes dry. Resident may have trouble swallowing

- Tongue becomes thick and coated

- Skin becomes dry, itching, or cracks

- Urine output decreases

- Urine is darker and cloudy

- Resident may be tired

- Confusion and mental impairment may develop

Edema

Edema may occur as the result of poor circulation, heart or kidney disease. Edema is swelling or the retention of fluid in the tissues. The nursing assistant must be alert for signs of edema in the residents. The indications of edema are the following:

- Swelling or puffiness, usually in feet, ankles, hands
- Difficulty breathing
  - Congestion or cough
  - Wheezing when breathing
- Weight increase
- Decrease in urine output

Ways to Get Enough Fluids

You are in the best position to help the resident get enough fluids. Some points to remember are the following:

- Refer to care plan. Know which fluids are restricted or encouraged. Some may be given between meals

- Offer fluids often, especially in hot weather or when resident has a fever

- Keep water fresh and nearby resident

- Record intake when indicated

- Help resident drink properly. Hold glass and straw if necessary

- Encourage resident to help himself. Use hand-on-hand technique or adaptive cups

- Record accurately all fluids on Intake and Output sheet

Helping with Meals

You will be responsible for helping the resident eat. This may include feeding the resident. You have already learned there are many factors that affect the resident's overall nutrition. Making mealtime pleasant and enjoyable should be the staff members' goal. Some ways to make mealtime pleasant are the following:

- Pleasant environment
  - Most residents will eat their meals in the dining room
  - If resident stays in his or her room, make the area clean and neat. Make it pleasant by removing objectionable items such as commodes, bedpans, urinals, etc.

- Social concerns
  - Ask residents where and with whom they wish to eat, if consistent with care plan
  - If facility permits it, encourage resident's family to eat a meal with them sometimes
  - Realize that the resident may feel resentment or be embarrassed if unable to feed himself

- Resident's comfort
  - Be sure that resident is clean and has recently toileted
  - Dress resident in comfortable clothing
  - Be certain resident is wearing dentures, eye glasses, and hearing aid at mealtime

- Proper positioning

- Adaptive equipment to allow self-feeding, if possible (Figure 10-2)
  - Plate guards
  - Adaptive silverware
  - Special cups, glasses

- Make sure residents are served the right tray

- Make sure foods are not too hot or too cold

- Notice and report resident's likes, dislikes, and techniques that do and do not help the resident meet nutritional needs

Feeding Techniques

Some techniques and methods to remember when feeding residents include the following:

- Proper positioning is important to prevent choking

- Prepare food according to resident's needs
  - Ask resident what you can do to help, such as cut meat, open cartons, etc.

- Encourage self-care
  - Let the resident feed himself foods that can be handled easily

- Use adaptive equipment

- Tell resident which items are hot

- Use clock description for the vision-impaired resident. For example meat on plate is at twelve o'clock location

- Check temperatures of foods before feeding

- Explain what foods are on tray. Ask the resident what he would like to eat first

- Feed residents that are unable to feed themselves

- Use hand-on-hand technique to help the resident

- Make sure resident swallows food before giving more

- Offer liquids at intervals

- Use a straw or spout cup for liquids

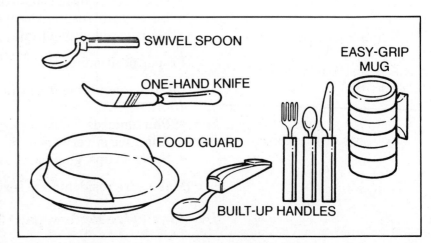

FIGURE 10-2.
Adaptive devices are used to help residents eat.

- Make pleasant conversation but do not ask the resident questions that take a long time to answer

- Never rush the resident

- Usually sitting next to resident conveys a nonrush feeling

- Sit at or below eye level to prevent the resident from bending head backwards, which may cause choking

Procedure 20

Feeding the Resident

1. Wash your hands.

2. Explain to resident who you are and what you are going to do.

3. Offer resident help with toileting.

4. Position resident in comfortable sitting position in bed or chair.

5. Position over-bed table over resident's lap.

6. Check meal tray for silverware, spilled foods.

7. Gather adaptive equipment, if necessary: napkin or towel, long-handled spoon, plate guard, or non-spill cup, etc.

8. Make sure it is the correct menu for the resident.

9. Place tray on table. Remove food covers.

10. Sit near resident.

11. Explain what is on tray.

12. Ask resident what foods he would like to eat first.

13. Encourage resident to feed himself, if able, by using finger foods or adaptive equipment.

14. Use hand-on-hand technique to help resident to feed himself.

15. Fill fork or spoon only half full or less, according to resident's ability to swallow.

16. Use straw for liquids.

17. Encourage resident. Talk pleasantly. Do not rush resident.

18. Wipe resident's mouth.

19. Offer liquids between amounts of solid food.

20. Remove tray when resident is finished.

21. Wash resident's hands, if necessary.

22. Replace side rail if it is lowered.

23. Leave resident comfortable.

24. Place call light within resident's reach.

25. Note amount of food and fluids taken, according to facility procedure.

26. Wash your hands.

27. Record or report amounts of food and fluid taken in. Record percentage or fractions on intake and output sheet. Note resident's eating, chewing, and self-help ability.

(See Procedure Review, page 251)

Other Means of Nutrition

There may be times in the long-term care facility when you will help the nurse feed the resident in different ways. The nursing assistant does not usually give these types of feedings, but an understanding of the techniques will help you care for the resident.

A feeding tube is used for residents who cannot swallow or for those who have a lot of trouble swallowing (Figure 10-3). **Intravenous** feedings are sometimes used to add to the resident's nutrition. These types of tube or intravenous feedings are often used for residents who have had a stroke, cancer of the throat, or some other major problem and cannot eat.

Types of feeding tubes

- Nasogastric Tube (N/G tube)
  - a soft, plastic tube inserted into a nostril. Goes down the throat into the stomach
  - About 12 inches of the tube is left out at nose and is usually taped to side of nose
  - Give mouth care often
  - Inserted only by nurse

- Gastrostomy Tube
  - A surgical procedure performed by the doctor
  - A tube is placed into the stomach through an opening made in the abdominal wall
  - About 8 inches of tube is left outside the body

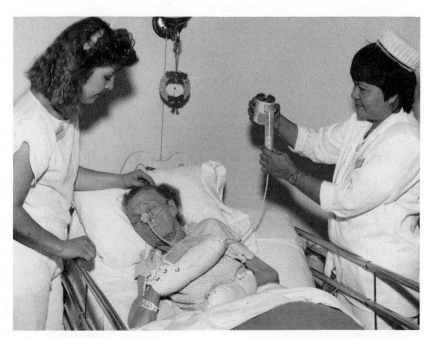

FIGURE 10-3.
The resident may be given proper nutrients through a feeding tube.

Safety Precautions When Caring for Resident Who has a Feeding Tube

- Never pull or tug on tubing. Keep resident from lying on tubing

- Keep the skin area around tube clean
  - Nasogastric tube
    - Clean nose around tube
    - Tube is usually taped at the nose
    - The end of the tubing is pinned to resident's clothing to prevent pulling
  - Gastrostomy
    - Clean skin area around tube
    - A clean gauze is often placed around at wound opening

- Report to the nurse immediately if
  - Alarm used to monitor feeding solution goes off
  - Tube becomes dislodged
  - Resident begins to cough, choke, or vomit
  - Feeding solution is not flowing properly
  - Feeding is leaking around gastrostomy tube
  - Skin is irritated around gastrostomy tube

- Refer to care plan for special instructions

Safety Precautions When Caring for a Resident Who has an Intravenous Line

- Refer to resident's care plan

- Make sure intravenous fluid is flowing

- Handle carefully the arm or leg of infusion site

- Do not adjust clamps on tubing

- Be careful when changing resident's gown

- Report to nurse immediately if
  - Swelling, redness, pain, or bleeding is at site of needle insertion
  - Fluid is not dripping
  - Level of fluid in bag is low or empty
  - Alarm used to monitor intravenous feeding goes off
  - Needle or tubing becomes dislodged

Intake and Output

Intake and Output is a procedure in which all liquids taken in by the resident and all liquids put out by the resident are recorded (Figure 10-4). This procedure is done to monitor the fluid balance of the resident. In most cases recording intake and output is the nursing

FIGURE 10-4.
Example of Intake and Output Record.

DAILY INTAKE AND OUTPUT RECORD
(Bedside record)

Intake   Output

11-7

Time	Oral	IV			Time	Urine	Emesis	Drainage	

Total:_____   Total:_____

7-3

Time	Oral	IV			Time	Urine	Emesis	Drainage	

Total:_____   Total:_____

3-11

Time	Oral	IV			Time	Urine	Emesis	Drainage	

Total:_____   Total:_____

Water glass	= 150 ml	Milk carton	= 240 ml
Coffee pot	= 200 ml	Large paper cup	= 240 ml
Ice cream	= 60 ml	(like for eggnog,	
Coffee cup	= 120 ml	shakes, etc.)	
Soup bowl	= 180 ml	Jello per serving	= 120 ml

assistant's responsibility. Intake and Output is abbreviated in most facilities as **I&O**. Some points relating to intake and output are the following:

- Explain the procedure to the resident. Request the resident's cooperation, if resident is able

- Record information accurately

- I&O sheets are often kept at the bedside

- Know facility policy on I&O. Usually amounts taken by resident are totaled at the end of each shift

Recording Intake

- Foods that are liquid at room temperature are recorded on I&O sheets

- Fluids from any source are recorded. The nurse records intravenous and tube feedings

- Record amounts under intake column in **cubic centimeters** (cc) or in **milliliters** (ml) according to facility policy

- Some measurements to be familiar with are the following:
  1 ounce equals 30 cc
  1 cup (8 oz) equals 240 cc
  1 teaspoon equals 4 cc

- The nursing assistant must learn the equivalents used in the facility. Most facilities provide conversion tables for recording intake

- Record only the amount actually taken by the resident. For example, do not record a full glass of water if resident drank only half of the glass.

Recording Output

- Output includes all fluids lost from the body
  - urine
  - blood or drainage
  - emesis (vomiting)
  - diarrhea
  - sweat

- Measured output by pouring urine or other discharge into a graduate (measuring pitcher). Record the amount shown on the pitcher

- If resident is incontinent, follow facility policy for recording urinary output

- Report to nurse immediately any blood or wound drainage

- Report excessive perspiration

- Record output under appropriate column on I&O sheet

Procedure 21

Recording Intake and Output

1. Wash your hands.

2. Explain to resident who you are and what you are going to do.

3. Check to identify equivalents used in your facility (e.g. coffee cup (5 oz) = 150 cc, glass (8 oz) = 240 cc).

4. Identify foods taken by resident that are considered liquid.

5. Estimate the amount of liquid food taken.

6. Record on I&O sheet in cubic centimeters the amount of liquid foods taken by resident.

7. Record amounts under intake column.

8. Measure output of resident by pouring contents of urinal, bedpan, or emesis basin into graduate (measuring pitcher).

9. Record the output in cubic centimeters in the appropriate column.

10. Leave resident comfortable and safe with call light within resident's reach.

11. Wash your hands.

12. Return meal tray to appropriate area.

13. Report or record, as indicated by facility policy.

(See Procedure Review, page 253)

Key Points in This Chapter

🔑 A balanced diet containing the essential nutrients is necessary to good health.

🔑 Many residents in the long-term care facility need some help getting proper nutrition.

🔑 Many residents will be on special diets. Make sure the resident receives the right tray at mealtime.

🔑 Fluid balance occurs when fluid intake and fluid output are about equal.

🔑 Dehydration occurs when there is not enough fluid in the body.

🔑 Making mealtime as pleasant as possible is the responsibility of the entire staff in the long-term care facility.

🔑 Let residents feed themselves whenever possible.

🔑 Be alert to safety when caring for residents who have feeding tubes.

🔑 When the resident is on I&O all liquids taken in must be recorded. Also, all liquid output must be measured and recorded.

Review Quiz Chapter 10
Nutritional and Fluid Needs

Choose the best answer for the questions below.

1. What are the four food groups?

   Ⓐ Meats, milk products, cereals, and fish
   Ⓑ Meats, milk products, bread, vegetables and fruits
   Ⓒ Milk products, meats, fish, fruits, and vegetables
   Ⓓ Milk products, meats, fish, cereals, and bread

2. What is the daily normal fluid intake for an adult?

   Ⓐ 1 quart
   Ⓑ 1 to 2 quarts
   Ⓒ 2 to 3 quarts
   Ⓓ More than 3 quarts

3. Which of the following statements is true?

   Ⓐ Proper nutrition can be obtained by eating proper amounts from the food groups.
   Ⓑ Everyone should take a vitamin pill every day.
   Ⓒ The elderly should take extra vitamin tablets at least once a week.
   Ⓓ Foods do not contain vitamins or minerals.

4. Which factors affect the resident's nutrition?

   Ⓐ Sensory loss
   Ⓑ General health
   Ⓒ Physical comfort
   Ⓓ All of the above

5. Which of the following are some ways the nursing assistant can help the resident at mealtime?

   Ⓐ Make sure the resident is dressed in comfortable clothing.
   Ⓑ Help the resident to a comfortable position for eating.
   Ⓒ Remove the resident's dentures before eating.
   Ⓓ All of the above
   Ⓔ A and B only

6. Cultural influences that may affect the eating habits of the resident are

   Ⓐ religion and family customs.
   Ⓑ proper fitting dentures.
   Ⓒ ability to chew or swallow.
   Ⓓ sensory loss.

7. Making mealtime a pleasant experience is the responsibility of

   Ⓐ the nursing assistant only.
   Ⓑ the dietary staff only.
   Ⓒ the housekeeping staff.
   Ⓓ all of the facility's staff.

8. Who is the person responsible for planning the meals for the resident?

   Ⓐ The resident
   Ⓑ The dietician
   Ⓒ The head nurse
   Ⓓ The administrator

9. Which of the following would *not* be included on a clear liquid diet?

   Ⓐ Tea
   Ⓑ Milk
   Ⓒ Broth
   Ⓓ Gelatin (Jello)

10. When serving a tray to a resident who must have a diabetic diet, you should make sure

   (A) there is no salt on the tray.
   (B) the resident does not have coffee.
   (C) there is no sugar on tray.
   (D) the tray has no fruit or vegetables on it.

11. Some residents must have a low-salt diet. A food that is high in salt content is

   (A) ham.
   (B) milk.
   (C) bread.
   (D) fruit.

12. Dehydration occurs when

   (A) there is too much fat in the body.
   (B) there is not enough fluid in the body.
   (C) one has overeaten.
   (D) the body is at rest.

13. When feeding a resident

   (A) turn on your favorite television program.
   (B) feed the resident all liquids before giving any solid foods.
   (C) be sure to avoid rushing the resident.
   (D) make sure all foods are room temperature.

14. A feeding tube may be inserted for residents

   (A) who cannot swallow.
   (B) who must have only liquids.
   (C) who are on a salt-restricted diet.
   (D) who have poorly fitted dentures.

15. When a resident is on Intake and Output, you must record

   (A) all the food the resident eats.
   (B) the liquids the resident has.
   (C) all the liquids served to the resident.
   (D) both the liquids and the solid food taken by the resident.

ANSWERS

1. B	6. A	12. B
2. C	7. D	13. C
3. A	8. B	14. A
4. D	9. B	15. B
5. E	10. C	
	11. A	

151

Chapter 11

Elimination Needs

In this chapter you will learn how to help the resident with elimination needs. After reading this chapter you should be able to:

- Define Key Terms
- Describe Normal Elimination
- Describe Factors which Interfere with Normal Elimination
- Describe Bowel and Bladder Management Guidelines
- Test Urine for Sugar and Acetone
- Position a Resident on a Bedpan
- Perform Catheter Care
- Describe Ostomy Care
- Identify Guidelines for Enema Administration

Key Terms

Anus: The opening of the rectum

Bowel: Same as intestine, part of the digestive system extending from the stomach to the rectum

Bedpan: A special shaped container to be used for bedridden residents to discharge body waste

Catheter: A tube inserted into a body cavity; often inserted into the bladder to drain urine

Colon: The large bowel; the lower part of the intestine

Commode: A portable toilet

Colostomy: A surgically created opening into the abdominal wall through which feces pass out of the body

Defecate: To have a bowel movement

Enema: Injection of fluid into the rectum; usually given to clean out the bowel

Feces: Waste products from the bowel, same as stool or bowel movement

Homeostasis: A constant state of balance within the body

Impaction: Mass of hard feces that cannot be passed from the rectum normally

Incontinent: Unable to control the passage of urine or stool

Involuntary: Done without choice; refers most often to inability to control stool passage

Ostomy: A surgically created opening through the abdominal wall into the intestines; body waste passes through this opening

Stoma: The opening on the abdomen created by an ostomy

Stool: Feces or bowel movement

Urethra: The body tube through which urine passes from the body

Urinate: To pass urine

Urinal: A container used by males to urinate into

Void: To pass urine

Normal Elimination

Elimination is the body's way of removing waste products and toxic substances through the digestive and genitourinary systems. A review of each of these body systems follows:

Genitourinary System

The genitourinary system eliminates waste products from the blood, forms urine, and allows for the discharge of urine. The genitourinary system is very important in maintaining **homeostasis**, or stable body function.

The organs in the genitourinary system are the following:

- Kidneys
  - Filter the blood
  - Return necessary water and chemicals to the blood after filtering out waste
  - Form urine from waste products taken from the blood

- Bladder
  - Stores the urine in a hollow sac until it is passed from the body

- Ureter
  - Tube that connects the kidneys to bladder

- Urethra
  - Tube through which urine passes out of body

Characteristics of normal urine are the following:
  - Clear or yellow golden colored

- Nearly odorless but smells like ammonia upon standing
- Free from sediment or mucous
- Urge to urinate is usually felt when bladder has 250-500 cc

Digestive System

In the digestive system, food is chemically broken down so it can be absorbed by the blood as nutrients.

The organs of the digestive system are the following:

- Mouth
  - Food is chewed and mixed with saliva

- Esophagus
  - Tube connecting mouth to stomach

- Stomach
  - Muscular organ where food is churned and mixed with digestive juices

- Intestines
  - Large and small tube-like canals that extend from the stomach to the rectum
  - Blood absorbs nutrients as food passes through the intestines
  - Undigested food is passed on as **stool (feces)** into the rectum

- The rectum
  - The last 5-6 inches of the colon
  - Feces are stored in the rectum until the urge to move bowels is felt

- Characteristics of normal feces are the following:
  - Light to dark brown color
  - Soft and formed
  - Frequency varies from daily bowel movement to every 3 days
  - No difficulty in passing normal stool

Interference with Normal Elimination _____

When caring for the elderly residents, you must be aware of things that can cause elimination problems (Figure 11-1). Some of these include:

- Aging
  - Normal aging slows down all body functions including those of the digestive and urinary systems
  - Feeling thirsty decreases with age. Many elderly do not take enough liquids to allow for proper elimination
  - Blood flow to kidneys is decreased so the genitourinary system functions less often

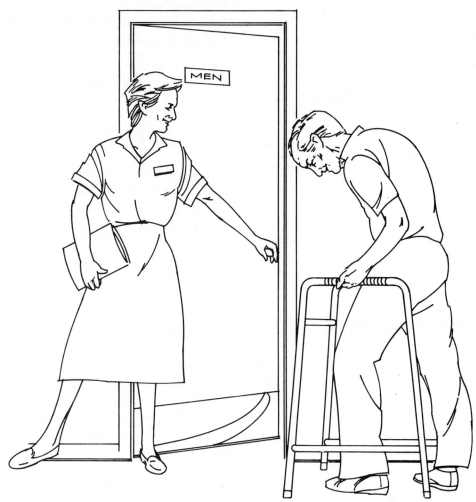

FIGURE 11-1.
Nursing assistants must be
aware of the resident's
toileting needs.

- Feeling of a full bladder and bowel is reduced. Elderly resident often feels urgency at the same time the feeling of elimination is felt

○ Disease and disability
  - Many residents have chronic illnesses that affect elimination
  - Residents may have nerve damage. This causes limited,
    reduced, or no feelings of urgency

○ Inactivity
  - The elimination systems rely on the stimulation from muscle
    movements to function effectively

○ Medication
  - Many residents take medicines that affect the elimination
    systems. Medication may cause diarrhea, constipation, or
    urinary problems
  - Many elderly persons have a history of taking laxatives.
    Laxatives affect normal intestinal function

○ Improper diet
  • Inadequate fluid intake can cause elimination problems
  • Food should have sufficient bulk or roughage

○ Lack of privacy
  • Many persons need privacy to have normal elimination

○ Stress
  • This emotion may cause diarrhea, constipation, or urinary frequency

○ Abnormal body position
  • Using a **bedpan** often is difficult
  • When resident remains in bed, urine tends to pool, making **voiding** difficult. This often leads to urinary tract infections

○ Time
  • A sufficient amount of time is needed

Bowel and Bladder Management

Many residents can relearn to control urine and stool passage. Bowel and bladder training plans take time and attention of all the nursing staff. A plan to retrain may require scheduling changes as well as a lot of effort from the nursing assistant. Once the process is relearned, however, it will become part of the daily routine and will save you time and energy.

The resident, of course, benefits from any bowel and bladder plan. Control of one's body functions adds to self-esteem, dignity, happiness, and health. Some points to remember in a bowel and bladder management plan are the following:

○ Establish regularity and prevent **incontinence**

○ Set plans according to each resident's pattern

○ Explain the procedure to the resident. It will ensure resident cooperation

○ Refer to care plan about
  • fluid intake
  • recording fluid output
  • positioning the resident
  • schedule of voiding intervals

○ Always report and record observations

○ Treat incontinence in a "matter-of-fact" manner. Never scold, yell at, or ridicule resident

Special Guidelines for Toileting

• Some residents cannot tell you they need to use the toilet. They may become restless or irritable instead

- Loss of appetite and small, watery rectal discharge may indicate a fecal **impaction**. Report to nurse immediately

- Pressure or full feeling in lower abdomen may indicate a full bladder or hard fecal mass. Report to nurse immediately

- The urge to eliminate may occur quickly and suddenly. Respond promptly

- Many residents must void more often at night

Help with Elimination Needs

Some of the ways you will help the resident with elimination needs will include helping the resident to the bathroom or helping the resident to the commode (Figure 11-2). A **commode** is a portable toilet. You will also be giving the resident the **bedpan** or **urinal**. These are specially shaped containers designed to help the bedridden resident urinate or defecate (Figure 11-3). Other duties you will perform are observing and reporting unusual output, providing catheter care, assisting with care for an ostomy and giving enemas. Information about these skills and the procedures to follow are listed below.

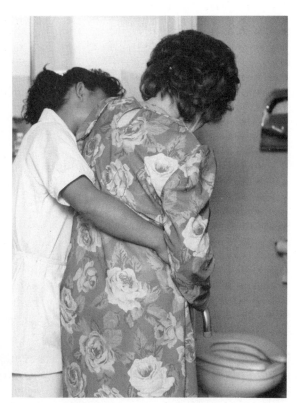

FIGURE 11-2.
Help the resident to the bathroom when necessary.

157

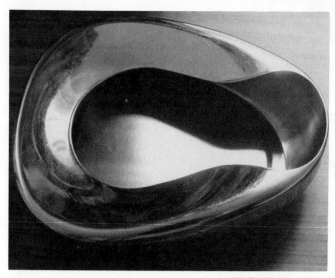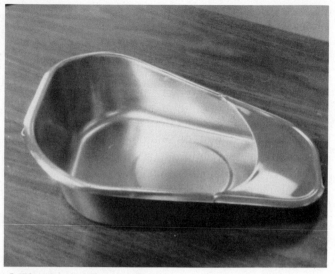

FIGURE 11-3a and Figure 11-3b.
Two types of bedpans: standard (left) and fracture (right).
The fracture bedpan is lower and is easier to position under the resident.

Procedure 22

Giving a Bedpan

1. Wash your hands.

2. Explain to resident who you are and what you are going to do.

3. Gather supplies: bedpan, bedpan cover, and tissue.

4. Give privacy.

5. Raise bed to working height. Lower head of bed.

6. Lower side rail on working side.

7. Fold upper linen down to expose resident's buttocks.

8. Place your hands on resident's shoulder and hip. Log roll (turn with resident's body in a straight line) resident to side away from you. Resident may help to turn by grasping side rail away from you. *Or,* ask resident to bend legs and raise buttocks.

9. Place bedpan so wider end of pan is aligned with resident's buttocks.

10. Hold pan in place while turning resident onto back if resident has been turned to side.

11. Cover resident.

12. Raise side rail.

13. Lower bed. Raise headrest unless resident must remain flat.

14. Place call light and tissue within reach of resident.

15. Leave room. Assure the resident's privacy.

16. Return when called by resident.

17. Gather supplies, if necessary, to clean perineal area of resident: gloves, basin of warm water, washcloth, and towel.

18. Lower head of bed. Raise bed to working level, lower side rail.

19. Fold covers back to expose resident's buttocks.

20. Turn resident on side away from you, place one hand on shoulder, and one hand on hip. *Or,* ask resident to bend legs and lift buttocks.

21. Hold bedpan while resident is turning or lifting.

22. Remove, cover, and place bedpan near foot of bed or on chair.

23. Put on gloves to wipe perineal area.

24. Clean perineal area with toilet tissue, if resident is unable.

25. Wash perineal area with warm, wet washcloth.

26. Rinse and dry perineal area very well.

27. Check skin for redness or irritation.

28. Turn resident to back.

29. Cover resident.

30. Position resident comfortably.

31. Raise side rail. Lower bed.

32. Empty contents of bedpan into toilet or graduate (measuring pitcher).

33. If resident is on I&O, measure urine.

34. Clean bedpan. Cover it and replace to proper area.

35. Wash your hands.

36. Help resident wash his hands.

37. Leave resident comfortable and safe.

38. Place call light within resident's reach.

39. Record or report output. Note color, amount, or anything unusual. Record condition of resident's skin.

(See Procedure Review, page 255)

Observing and Measuring Output of Resident

- Urine
  - Measure and record in cubic centimeters, or millimeters, as indicated by facility policy
  - If the resident is **incontinent**, (unable to control the passage of urine) follow facility procedure by measuring size of urine puddle or weight of pad
  - Record amounts in drainage bags by measuring in graduate

- Feces (bowel movements)
  - Recording is extremely important to ensure elimination is adequate
  - Most facilities use check-list charting for recording bowel movements

- Observe and report anything unusual in stool or urine
  - Blood

- Mucous
- Liquid stool
- Very hard stool
- Undigested food or pills in stool

○ Intake and output sheet (I&O)
- Record amount of urine
- Note profuse perspiration or sweat
- Note time of output, if required

○ Record on output sheet any amount of vomit (emesis)

Testing Urine for Sugar and Acetone

You may be assigned to test the resident's urine for sugar and acetone. This procedure is done for the diabetic resident. **Diabetes** is a disease in which the body does not make enough insulin. Insulin is made by the body and is necessary to break down carbohydrates. Remember that carbohydrates are a necessary food nutrient.

When a resident has diabetes, these carbohydrates or sugars are not used properly by the body. The carbohydrates are eaten by the resident, digested, and then absorbed by the blood. The blood goes through the kidneys, which gets rid of the extra carbohydrates (sugar) into the urine. Testing the urine is a simple way to find out how much sugar is in the blood. Acetones or ketones also are found in urine when carbohydrates are not used correctly by the body.

Several methods may be used to test urine for sugar and acetone. Always refer to the instructions on the bottle when using any product for testing urine. For each test you will be using a reagent, a chemical substance. General rules for urine tests are the following:

- Do procedure at correct time

- Always use a fresh urine specimen

- Make sure you have clean equipment: bedpan, urinal or specimen container

- Keep reagent tablets or strips dry. Keep lid on tight and equipment in safe place. Tablets and strips are poisonous

- Follow instructions on container for use

- Wear gloves

- Know and follow the facility policy

- Be accurate in reading test and timing reactions. The amount of medication the resident receives may be based on your recording

- Report or record findings to the nurse

Catheters

A **catheter** is a tube inserted into a body cavity, usually for the purpose of draining liquids. The most commonly used catheter is the urinary catheter, which is inserted by the nurse. Often the catheter is an in-dwelling tube. That is, a tube that stays in the bladder for a period of time (Figure 11-4). The in-dwelling catheter has a small balloon inflated after placement in the bladder. The catheter is attached to tubing that connects to a drainage bag, which collects the urine.

Catheter Care

This procedure may vary from one facility to another. Always refer to care plan for specific instructions. Some general guidelines do apply to catheter care. They include the following:

- Maintain cleanliness
  - Gently wash genital area around catheter with warm water
  - Wash perineal area. Wash from front to back on females
  - Rinse and dry very well

- Make sure tubing is without kinks

- Make sure all connections are tight

- Make sure resident is not lying or sitting on tubing

- Check care plan to see whether catheter should be positioned to prevent pulling on the bladder
  - For females, catheter may be taped to upper thigh
  - For males, catheter may be taped horizontally to the thigh or on the abdomen

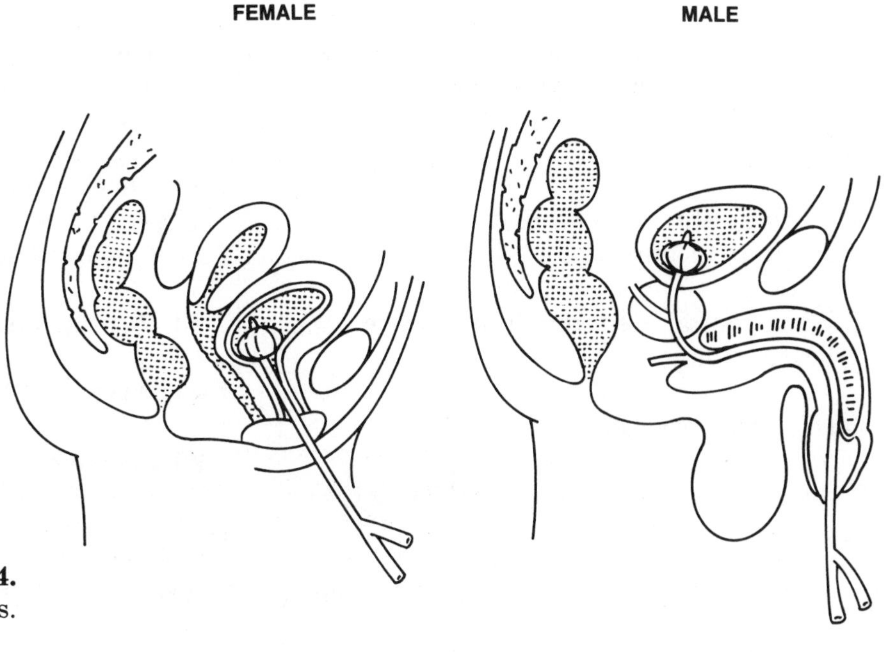

FEMALE   MALE

FIGURE 11-4.
Placement of in-dwelling catheters.

○ Attach drainage tubing to sheet to let urine drain well

○ Lower drainage bag below level of bladder at all times. Urine drains from bladder by gravity

○ Attach drainage bag to bed frame, not side rail

○ Never pull or put tension on catheter or tubing

○ Use care when moving residents with catheters, be alert to tubing position

○ Follow facility procedure when emptying drainage bag, record appropriately

Procedure **23**
Giving Catheter Care

1. Wash your hands.

2. Explain to resident who you are and what you are going to do.

3. Gather supplies: basin of warm water, washcloth, towel, gloves, tape or rubber band, and pin

4. Give privacy.

5. Raise bed to working height.

6. Lower side rail on working side.

7. Fold top linen down to expose catheter.

8. Observe tubing for urine flow, pressure, secure connections, and kinks.

9. Put on gloves.

10. Wash urethra area around catheter entrance (Figure 11-5).

11. Wash genital area from front area to back. Rinse often.

12. Dry area very well.

13. Secure or attach catheter, according to care plan.

14. Place drainage tubing over resident's leg.

15. Place tape or rubber band around tubing and pin tape or rubber band to sheet at edge of mattress to make sure that extra tubing stays on bed.

16. Cover resident.

17. Raise side rail. Lower bed.

18. Empty drainage bag. Open clamp on bag. Let urine drain into a graduate. This is usually done at end of shift.

19. Record amount of urine.

20. Make sure drainage bag is lower than bladder and attached securely to bed frame.

21. Check tubing to make sure urine is flowing.

22. Leave resident comfortable and safe.

23. Place call light within resident's reach.

24. Wash your hands.

25. Record or report output. Note color, amount, and anything unusual.

(See Procedure Review, page 259)

Ostomies

An **ostomy** is a surgical opening made through the abdomen to allow body waste to come out (Figure 11-6). This procedure is done when disease or injury prevents normal elimination. An ostomy may be done to allow for urinary or fecal waste discharge. The opening of the ostomy is called the **stoma**. Ostomies may be temporary or permanent. The most common type of ostomy is the colostomy, an opening into the colon to allow for feces to be eliminated. Many people live well with ostomies. They still work and are very active. The resident in a long-term care facility many need some assistance with caring for the ostomy. Procedures may vary from one facility to another. However, some general guidelines apply.

Caring for the Resident with an Ostomy

- Realize the resident with an ostomy may feel a great loss of control and have a poor body image and low self-esteem

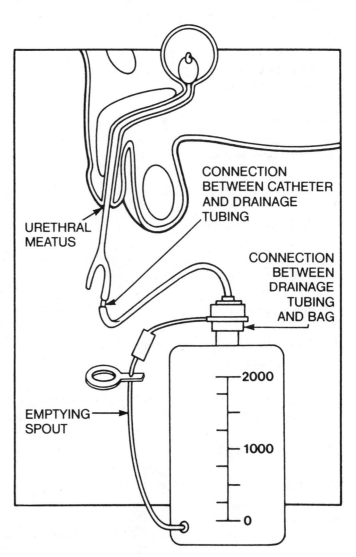

FIGURE 11-5.
Take special care to protect contamination sites of catheters.

- Be a good listener. Allow the resident to talk about his or her feelings

- Report to nurse signs of depression

- Wear gloves

- Wash area around ostomy

- Observe and report any changes in the skin around the stoma

- Apply protective cream around stoma, if indicated

- Change ostomy bags often to reduce odors

- Throw away soiled bags properly

Enemas

An **enema** is the injection of fluid into the rectum, usually done to empty the rectum of feces. You may be given the responsibility of giving a resident an enema. There are two types of enemas: a cleansing enema and a retention enema. The cleansing enema is given to clean out the rectum. The retention enema is given to soften the feces or to administer medication.

The type of enema nursing assistants usually administer is the cleansing enema. The solution for enemas may be plain water, a soap or salt solution, or a commercial preparation.

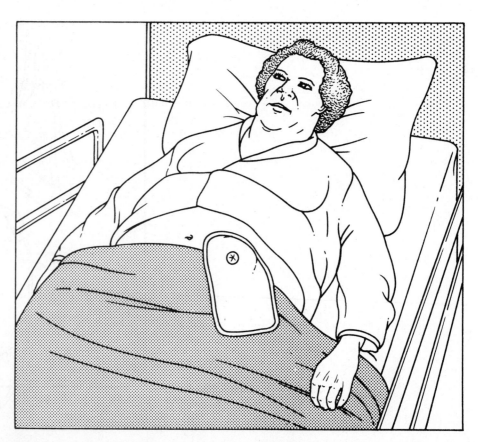

FIGURE 11-6.
An ostomy bag is in place on a resident's abdomen.

Policies of long-term care facilities will vary as to who is responsible for giving enemas. Check with the nurse before giving a resident an enema. Some general guidelines to observe when administering enemas are the following:

- Check with nurse about which solution to use

- Enema solution should be warm, about 105 degrees

- Amount of solution should be 700 to 1000 cc (less than one quart)

- Have resident's bathrobe, bedpan, or commode nearby. Resident will feel urgency after enema

- Wear gloves

- Resident should be lying on left side

- Always lubricate the rectal tube of the enema

- Before inserting tubing into the rectum clear air from tubing by running water through tubing. Clamp tubing

- Insert tube about 3 to 4 inches

- Raise container of solution 12 to 18 inches over rectum

- Allow solution to run into rectum slowly

- If resident has cramping, clamp the tubing quickly a couple of times

- Tell resident to take deep breaths to ease cramping

- Give amount of solution ordered or as tolerated by resident

- Ask resident to hold solution in rectum for a few minutes, if possible

- Help resident to bathroom, commode, or onto bedpan

- Make sure resident's call light is within reach

- Observe and report the results of the enema. Instruct resident not to flush toilet until results have been observed

Key Points in This Chapter

🔑 Elimination of body waste is done through the body's digestive and genitourinary systems.

🔑 Due to reduced sensitivity, the elderly person will often have a sense of urgency at the same time the void is felt.

🔑 Some factors affecting normal elimination in the resident may be disease, inactivity, medications, and lack of privacy.

🔑 Bowel and bladder management programs can help the resident regain control over these body functions.

🔑 Testing urine for sugar and acetone may be done for the resident who has diabetes.

🔑 Catheter care includes cleaning the genital area and watching for proper urine drainage.

🔑 Enemas are the injection of fluid into the rectum, usually done to remove feces.

🔑 An ostomy is an opening into the abdomen to allow body waste to come out.

Review Quiz Chapter 11
Elimination needs

Choose the best answer for the questions below.

1. The body's way of removing waste products is called

   Ⓐ digestion.
   Ⓑ circulation.
   Ⓒ elimination.
   Ⓓ excretion.

2. The organ(s) of the urinary system that filter the blood and form urine is (are) the

   Ⓐ bowel.
   Ⓑ kidney.
   Ⓒ bladder.
   Ⓓ intestines.

3. Normal urine is

   Ⓐ clear.
   Ⓑ dark yellow.
   Ⓒ foul smelling.
   Ⓓ streaked with mucous.

4. What are intestines?

   Ⓐ Tubes connecting the kidneys and bladder
   Ⓑ Tube-like canals extending from stomach to rectum
   Ⓒ A storage place for urine before discharge
   Ⓓ The tubes through which blood circulates to the body

5. In normal aging, the blood flow to the kidneys is

   Ⓐ lessened.
   Ⓑ increased.
   Ⓒ stimulated.
   Ⓓ not changed.

6. Which of the following may be factors causing elimination problems in the elderly?

   Ⓐ Normal aging
   Ⓑ Improper diet
   Ⓒ Lack of activity
   Ⓓ All of the above

7. Bowel and bladder training plans should include

   Ⓐ the resident only.
   Ⓑ only the nursing staff on the night shift.
   Ⓒ the entire nursing staff involved with care of the resident.
   Ⓓ all of the administration staff of the facility.

8. All of the following statements are true *except*

   Ⓐ many residents will have the urge to urinate more frequently at night.
   Ⓑ the urge to eliminate will occur quickly and urgently in many residents.
   Ⓒ all residents will be unable to control the urine passage while sleeping.
   Ⓓ some residents may be restless and irritable, which may indicate a need to eliminate urine.

9. What does the term void mean?

   Ⓐ To pass stool
   Ⓑ To pass urine; to urinate
   Ⓒ To insert a tube to drain urine
   Ⓓ To end the passage of urine or stool

10. When placing a resident on a bedpan,

   (A) make certain resident has privacy.
   (B) make certain resident is positioned on bedpan properly.
   (C) place the call light within resident's reach.
   (D) All of the above

11. After removing a bedpan from a resident, you noticed some blood in the urine. What is your best response?

   (A) Empty bedpan, and clean and replace equipment.
   (B) Empty bedpan into toilet, then record the incident on the resident's chart.
   (C) Place bedpan and contents in bathroom. Report appearance of blood in urine to nurse immediately.
   (D) Save urine in container and send it to the doctor's office for examination.

12. A nursing assistant may be asked to test the diabetic resident's urine for

   (A) blood.
   (B) alcohol.
   (C) proteins.
   (D) sugar and acetone.

13. Caring for the resident with a urinary catheter includes

   (A) making sure the tube has no kinks.
   (B) inserting the catheter into the resident.
   (C) removing the catheter at night.
   (D) changing the catheter every other day.

14. An opening made through the abdomen to allow for discharge of body waste is a(n)

   (A) enema.
   (B) ostomy.
   (C) catheter.
   (D) defecation.

15. When placing a resident on a commode to defecate, you are

   (A) helping the resident to sit on a bedpan.
   (B) helping the resident use a portable toilet to urinate.
   (C) placing the resident on a portable toilet to have a bowel movement.
   (D) placing the resident on a bedpan to have a bowel movement.

ANSWERS
1. C
2. B
3. A
4. B
5. A
6. D
7. C
8. C
9. B
10. D
11. C
12. D
13. A
14. B
15. C

168

Chapter 12

Vital Signs

In this chapter you will learn how to accurately measure and record the vital signs of body temperature, pulse, respiration, and blood pressure. After reading this chapter you should be able to:

- Define Key Terms
- Describe Vital Signs
- Measure the Resident's Body Temperature, Pulse and Respirations
- Measure the Resident's Blood Pressure
- Identify Abnormal Vital Signs
- Record the Resident's Vital Signs

Key Terms

Axillary: Having to do with the armpit area

Blood pressure: The pressure of the blood against the walls of the blood vessels

Body temperature: The amount of heat in the body measured by a thermometer

Brachial pulse: Pulse felt on the inner side of the arm at bend of elbow

Cyanosis: A bluish color in the skin, lips, or fingertips due to a lack of oxygen

Diastolic pressure: The lower number of a blood pressure reading; the relaxing phase of the heart beat cycle

Dyspnea: Difficult breathing

Hypertension: Abnormally high blood pressure

Hypotension: Abnormally low blood pressure

Oxygen: A colorless, odorless gas necessary for human life

Oral: Having to do with the mouth

Pulse: The beat of the heart as felt through the walls of the arteries

Radial pulse: Pulse felt at radial artery on the inner side of the wrist

Respiration: The exchange of oxygen and carbon dioxide in the body

Sphygmomanometer: The cuff used when taking blood pressure

Systolic pressure: The top number of the blood pressure reading; the contraction phase of the heart cycle

Vital signs: The temperature, pulse, respirations, and blood pressure

Vital Signs

The **vital signs** measure the functions of vital organs of the body (Figure 12-1). These four functions are temperature, pulse, respiration, and blood pressure. All are necessary for life. When the body is not functioning normally the rates and character of vital signs change. The resident's condition can be monitored and evaluated by measuring the vital signs.

It is extremely important that you know how to correctly take and accurately record vital signs. Whenever you are not sure of the readings, tell the nurse immediately. Accurate measurement of the vital signs takes learning and practice.

Abbreviations for vital signs

You must become familiar with the commonly used abbreviations for the vital signs. They are:

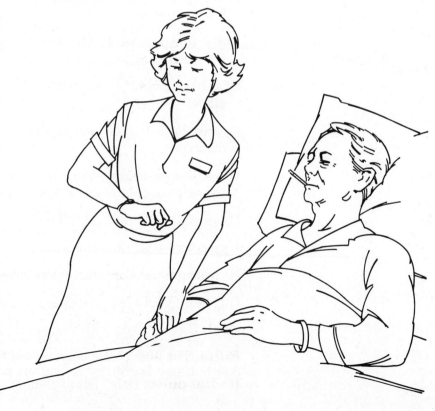

FIGURE 12-1.
Accuracy is very important when taking vital signs.

BP - Blood pressure

VS - Vital signs

TPR - Temperature, pulse and respiration

O - Oral temperature (taken in the mouth)

R - Rectal temperature (taken in the rectum)

A or Ax - Axillary temperature (taken in the axilla or armpit)

F - Fahrenheit measurement

C - Centigrade or Celsius measurement

Temperature

The **temperature** measures body heat. Body heat is created by food changing into energy. Body heat is lost by evaporation, respiration, and excretion. The balance between the heat produced by the body and the heat lost is the body temperature.

The normal aging process may interfere with the body's ability to regulate the temperature. Careful temperature monitoring is important for the resident in a long-term care facility. Other factors that might affect the body temperature are the following:

- o Body temperature can be increased by
  - Infection, illness, and disease
  - Dehydration
  - Physical exercise
  - Intake of hot liquids
  - Very warm environment

- o Body temperature can be decreased by
  - Shock
  - Cold environment
  - Medications

Thermometers

The temperature of the resident is taken using a thermometer. There are several types of thermometers: glass, electronic, plastic, and paper. The glass or electronic thermometers are most commonly used. Follow your facility's policy when using plastic or paper thermometers.

Thermometers measure body temperature using either Fahrenheit or Celsius scales (Figure 12-2). Both scales are divided into units called degrees. Check which type of thermometer your facility uses.

On glass thermometers, each long line on the thermometer equals one degree and each short line equals two tenths of a degree. The thermometer is read by noting the point at which the red mercury col-

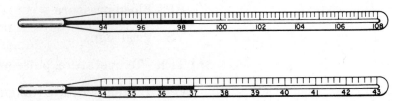

FIGURE 12-2.
Top thermometer has Fahrenheit scale;
lower thermometer has Celsius scale.

umn ends. The temperature is read to the nearest two tenths of a degree.

The electronic thermometer is a battery-operated unit that tells you the temperature reading on a lighted display. This type of unit eliminates human error that may occur with other types of thermometers. The electronic unit can be used for oral, rectal, or axillary temperatures.

Disposable plastic sheath covers are inserted over the electronic probe. A clean probe must be used for each resident's temperature. A special probe, often colored red, is used for rectal temperatures. The batteries of electronic thermometers must be charged regularly to stay accurate. Follow your facility's policy when using the electronic thermometer.

Methods of Measuring Body Temperature

There are three methods of measuring a resident's body temperature. The **oral** method is done by inserting the thermometer under the resident's tongue. The **rectal** method is done by inserting the thermometer one inch into the resident's rectum. The **axillary** method is done by placing the thermometer in the resident's armpit. Always refer to the care plan to learn which method must be used for each resident. A brief overview of each of these methods follows:

- ○ Oral (taken by mouth)
  - Use when the resident is alert and cooperative
  - Oral thermometer may have a bulb or slender tip with mercury. Sometimes the end of the thermometer is colored blue or green
  - Do not take temperature by mouth if resident has just taken hot or cold liquids, just smoked a cigarette, or chewed gum. Wait 5 to 10 minutes before taking oral temperature
  - Follow universal precautions. Wear gloves, if indicated
  - Normal oral temperature is 98.6° F

- ○ Rectal (taken in the rectum)
  - Thermometer has a shorter, rounded bulb tip with mercury
  - The tip opposite the mercury end of the rectal thermometer is usually red
  - Use for residents receiving oxygen ("mouth breathers"), confused or disoriented residents, and others who cannot keep thermometer in mouth

- Wear gloves when taking rectal temperatures. Follow universal precautions principles
- Always lubricate thermometer before inserting into rectum
- Always hold thermometer in place when taking rectal temperature
- Normal rectal temp is 99.6° F
- Record "R" if temperature was taken rectally

○ Axillary
- Use oral thermometer
- Remove perspiration by wiping axillary area before placing thermometer
- Normal axillary temp is 97.6° F
- Record "A" or "Ax" when axillary temperature is taken

○ Realize "normal temperature" is a range of normal. Each resident has his own true normal. Elderly residents' temperature may be slightly lower

○ Always immediately report to nurse unusually high or low temperatures

Guidelines for Taking Temperature

- Check thermometer for chips and cracks

- Follow facility's procedure for wiping up broken thermometer. The mercury in the glass thermometer is poison

- Be alert to thermometers with both Celsius and Fahrenheit scales. The markings on this type of thermometer are very small. Be sure to read accurately

- Shake mercury down before inserting thermometer

- Use care when shaking down thermometer. Stand away from resident or surfaces that thermometer may hit

- Stay with resident when taking temperature

- Lubricate rectal thermometer before inserting

- Hold rectal thermometer in place

- Wipe thermometer from colored or stem end to mercury tip before inserting

- Disinfect thermometers according to facility policy

- Never clean mercury thermometer with hot water. The thermometer will break

- Use clean probe cover for each resident when using electronic thermometer

Pulse

The **pulse** is the expansion and contraction of an artery. This rhythmic expansion and contraction in the artery indicates how fast the heart is beating. The pulse tells you how well the circulatory system is working. When you are taking the resident's pulse be alert to the rate, rhythm, and volume of the pulse beat.

Pulse Rate

The pulse rate is the number of beats per minute. The pulse rate varies within individuals from time to time depending upon exercise or emotional state. The pulse should be counted while the resident is at rest. Some points to remember are the following:

- Pulse rate varies. It depends on age, sex, body size, emotional state and exercise

- Usually pulse rate goes up as body temperature increases

- Pain usually increases pulse rate

- Medications may affect pulse rate

- Average adult pulse rate is 60 - 80 beats per minute

- Terms
  - Tachycardia: fast pulse rate, usually over 100 beats per minute
  - Bradycardia: slow pulse rate, usually less than 60 beats per minute

An irregular pulse occurs when the beats have a regular, even beat mixed with uneven or even skipped beats. When taking the pulse you must report any unusual beats.

- Regular
  - The pulse beats are evenly spaced

- Irregular
  - The pulse beats are uneven or there are skipped beats

Pulse Volume

The pulse volume is the forcefulness or degree of strength of the pulse. The volume of the pulse can be measured indirectly as the amount of force the blood exerts on the artery when expanding and contracting. You will feel the pulse and note if it is:

- Strong

- Weak

- Thready

Pulse Location

- Radial
  - Felt at the wrist
  - Most commonly used to take pulse (Figure 12-3)

- Carotid
  - Felt at side of neck

- Apical
  - Felt at the base of the heart
  - A stethoscope must be used to take the apical pulse
  - Usually done by the nurse

- Brachial
  - Felt at innerside of arm at elbow bed

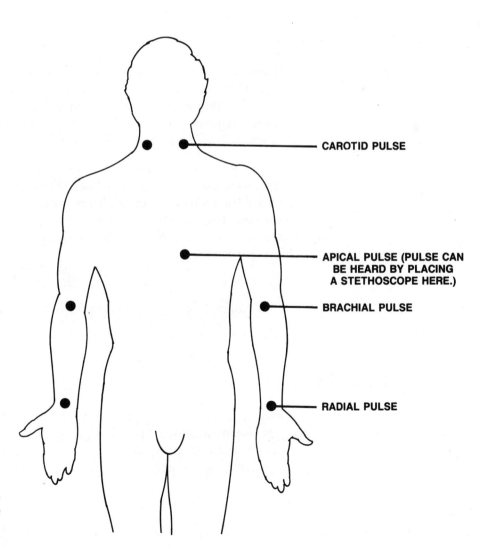

CAROTID PULSE

APICAL PULSE (PULSE CAN
BE HEARD BY PLACING
A STETHOSCOPE HERE.)

BRACHIAL PULSE

RADIAL PULSE

FIGURE 12-3.
Locations where
pulse can be felt.

Guidelines for Pulse Measurement

- Resident should be at rest

- Arm must rest on surface

- Use tips of 2 or 3 of your fingers. Never use thumb because you may feel your own pulse in your thumb

- Note rate—number of beats

- Note rhythm—regularity

- Note volume—weak, thready, strong

- Count for 30 seconds if pulse is regular. Count for 1 minute if pulse is irregular, or as indicated by your facility or on resident's care plan

- Record what pulse would be after 1 minute. If counting for 30 seconds, double the number and record it

- Report to nurse immediately if pulse is unusually fast, slow, or irregular

Respiration

Respiration is the process of breathing. It is this process which allows humans to take in **oxygen** and give off carbon dioxide. A single respiration or breath is one inspiration (breathing air in; inhaling) and one expiration (breathing air out; exhaling). As a nursing assistant you will be responsible for counting the resident's respirations.

The process of breathing is voluntary. That is, a person can control their respirations by holding their breath. This is the reason you do not explain to the residents that you are counting the respirations. Counting respirations usually is done after counting the pulse. The resident will think you are taking the pulse while you discreetly count the respirations.

Some factors relating to respiration are the following:

- Normal respirations for adults are 16 to 22 per minute

- Respirations increase with
  - infections
  - fever
  - emotional upsets or stress
  - exercise

- Respirations decrease with
  - some medications
  - some diseases

Guidelines Counting Respirations

○ Breathing can be controlled so the resident is not told when respirations are counted

○ One inspiration and one expiration of breath is counted as one respiration. Watch rise and fall of the resident's chest

○ Count respirations immediately after the pulse count. Remember the pulse count as you count the rise and fall of the chest

○ Keep your fingers in same position on wrist as when counting pulse

○ Note if respirations are
  • regular
  • shallow
  • deep
  • difficult or labored

○ Count respiration for 30 seconds or 1 minute as indicated by your facility or the resident's care plan

○ Count for 1 minute if respirations are irregular

○ Record what respirations would be for 1 minute. If counting for 30 seconds, double and record number

Blood Pressure

Measuring **blood pressure** gives valuable information about how the heart and blood vessels are working. The heart pumps the blood throughout the body through the arteries. The arteries carry blood away from the heart. When you take a resident's blood pressure, you are measuring how much pressure is exerted on the artery walls as the blood passes through. There is always some blood in the arteries, so there is always some pressure on the walls of these blood vessels. As the heart contracts to send out blood, a force is felt on the artery. This contracting time of the heart is called the **systolic pressure**. When the heart relaxes between beats, the pressure is lower. This is called the **diastolic pressure**. You will be reading both of these pressures when you take a blood pressure measurement.

The blood vessels of the older person are often thicker and less elastic, causing the heart to work somewhat harder to push blood through the arteries. For this reason, the blood pressure in the older resident is often higher than a normal adult's blood pressure.

Equipment Used to Measure Blood Pressure

The equipment used in measuring blood pressure varies from one facility to another. In all cases you will be using something called a **sphygmomanometer**, commonly referred to as a blood pressure cuff (Figure 12-4). Unless you are using a electronic digital recording

STETHOSCOPE

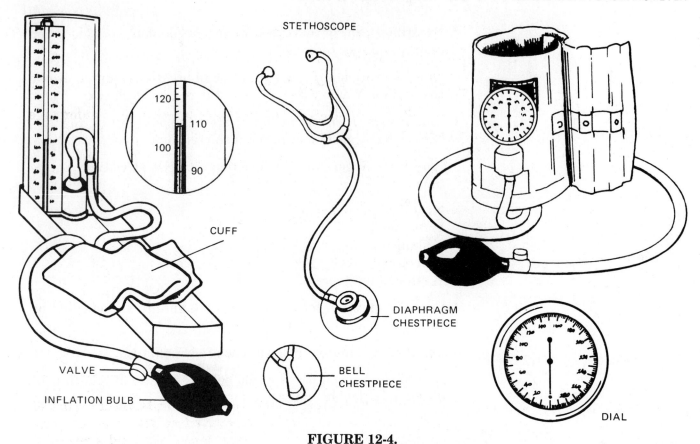

120
110
100
90

CUFF

DIAPHRAGM CHESTPIECE

BELL CHESTPIECE

VALVE

INFLATION BULB

DIAL

FIGURE 12-4.
Equipment used to measure blood pressure.

sphygmomanometer, you will also be using a stethoscope to listen to the reading. Equipment may be either

○ Mercury sphygmomanometer
  • A column of mercury is observed as you read the blood pressure

○ Aneroid sphygmomanometer
  • A pointer on a dial is observed as you read the blood pressure

Accuracy is very important in taking the blood pressure. It takes skill and practice to learn to take accurate blood pressure readings. Ask the nurse to recheck a reading if you are not sure.

Terms Associated with Blood Pressure

○ **Hypertension**
  • High blood pressure (usually 140/90 or higher)
  • Elderly person's blood pressure tends to be slightly higher than 140/90)

○ **Hypotension**
  • Low blood pressure (usually 98/70 or less)

Guidelines for Taking Blood Pressure

- Equipment should be in good working condition

- Use proper cuff size

- Have gauge at eye level

- Resident should be sitting or lying in a relaxed comfortable position, with arm resting on solid surface

- Use arm indicated on resident's care plan

- Do not use an arm
  - That has an intravenous infusion in it
  - That has been weakened by a stroke

- Inflate cuff to about 160 mm. If sound is heard upon immediate release of air, deflate cuff right away and reinflate to a higher number

- Record accurately in fraction form (120/80)

Recording Vital Signs

Recording vital signs you have measured is an important part of your role as a nursing assistant. Accuracy and writing in a clear way is necessary. Your facility may have you record the vital signs on a graphic sheet or on a daily flow sheet. You will learn procedures in your orientation to the facility. Ask for help if you are unsure of the method your facility uses.

Review Abbreviations for Vital Signs

- T - temperature

- P - pulse

- R - respiration

- BP - blood pressure

- VS - vital signs (includes all of above)

Proper way to Record

- List temperature first

- List count pulse second

- List respiration last
  - T   P   R
  - 98.6 - 80 - 20

○ Always write "R" behind temperature when temperature is taken rectally
  • 99.6R - 80 - 18

○ Always write "A" or "AX" behind temperature when temperature is taken axillary
  • 97.8A - 80 - 18

○ If temperature is not followed by a "R" or "A", the nurse will assume the temperature is an oral temperature reading

○ Write blood pressure as a fraction such as 120/80

○ Record accurately

○ Follow facility policy on recording vital signs

Procedure **24**

Taking the Oral Temperature

1. Wash your hands.

2. Explain to resident who you are and what you want to do.

3. Gather supplies: oral thermometer, watch with a second hand, pencil and paper, tissue, and gloves.

4. Rinse thermometer with cold water and wipe with tissue from stem to mercury bulb end, if thermometer has been in disinfectant.

5. Read thermometer. Shake down to 96°F.

6. Ask resident if he has had hot or cold liquids or smoked a cigarette. If so, wait 10 minutes.

7. Place bulb of thermometer under resident's tongue.

8. Ask resident to close lips and breathe through nose.

9. Note time of insertion and remove in 5 minutes or time interval on facility policy.

10. Wipe thermometer from stem to bulb with tissue.

11. Read thermometer to nearest two tenths of a degree.

12. Record temperature on paper.

13. Clean thermometer, if indicated, or replace in container.

14. Leave resident comfortable and safe.

15. Place call light within resident's reach.

16. Wash your hands.

17. Record on sheet according to facility policy.

18. Report any unusual temperature to nurse.

(See Procedure Review, page 261)

Procedure **25**

Taking the Pulse and Respirations

1. Wash your hands.

2. Explain to the resident who you are and what you want to do. Tell the resident you are taking the pulse. Do not tell resident you are going to count respirations.

3. Gather supplies: watch with a second hand, and pencil and paper.

4. Position resident's arm on flat surface. Ask resident to relax arm.

5. Place tips of 2 or 3 of your fingers on the palm and thumb side of resident's wrist.

6. Locate pulse with your fingers.

7. Do not use thumb to feel pulse.

8. Press lightly with fingers to feel pulse.

9. Look at the position of second hand on watch.

10. Count and remember the pulse beats for 30 seconds. Note volume and rhythm. Count for 1 minute, if pulse is irregular.

11. Continue to hold the resident's wrist as if you are still taking the pulse count.

12. Observe the rising and falling of the resident's chest.

13. Count one rise and one fall of chest as one respiration.

14. Count for 30 seconds. Note regularity. Count for 1 minute if respirations are irregular.

15. Remove your hand from resident's wrist.

16. Multiply by two the number of pulse beats, if counted for 30 seconds.

17. Record on paper the 1-minute pulse.

18. Multiply by two the number of respirations, if counted for 30 seconds.

19. Record on paper the 1-minute respirations.

20. Leave resident comfortable and safe.

21. Place call light within resident's reach.

22. Wash your hands.

23. Record on sheet according to facility policy.

24. Report any unusual findings to nurse.

(See Procedure Review, page 263)

Procedure 26

Taking the Blood Pressure

1. Wash your hands.

2. Explain to the resident who you are and what you want to do. Tell the resident this is not a painful procedure, but he or she may feel some tingling or numbness in arm.

3. Gather supplies: sphygmomanometer with proper cuff size, stethoscope, pencil and paper, and alcohol wipes.

4. Check earpieces of stethoscope. Clean with alcohol wipes.

5. Help resident to comfortable position in bed or chair.

6. Remove or loosen clothing from arm.

7. Place arm in comfortable position on flat surface.

8. Locate the brachial artery.

9. Make sure cuff is decompressed.

10. Wrap cuff snugly and smoothly around upper arm. Place it about one inch above bend of elbow. The inflatable portion of cuff must be over brachial artery.

11. Make sure tubing from cuff is centered.

12. Place earpieces of stethoscope in your ears.

13. Relocate the brachial artery.

14. Place diaphragm of stethoscope over brachial artery.

15. Hold stethoscope in place tightly against skin.

16. Tighten clockwise the thumb screw of valve on rubber bulb with other hand.

17. Squeeze rubber bulb to inflate the cuff and to raise dial of mercury to approximately 160-170 mm or as indicated on care plan.

18. Open thumb screw of valve just enough to hear air escape. Allow dial or mercury to slowly go down, dropping about 2 mm per beat.

19. Watch gauge carefully and listen for first clear sound of regular beats.

20. Read and remember column or dial number of the systolic reading.

21. Let air continue escaping slowly.

22. Listen carefully for the last sound.

23. Read and remember column or dial at this point for the diastolic reading.

24. Loosen thumb screw quickly and let all the air out of inflatable cuff.

25. Remove cuff from resident's arm.

26. Remove stethoscope from ears.

27. Record readings in fraction format on paper.

28. Leave resident comfortable and safe.

29. Place call light within resident's reach.

30. Clean earpieces of stethoscope with alcohol wipes.

31. Wash your hands.

32. Replace equipment.

33. Record on sheet according to facility policy.

34. Report any unusual findings to nurse.

(See Procedure Review, page 265)

Key Points in This Chapter

🔑 The vital signs tell you how well the body's vital organs are working.

🔑 The body temperature can be measured orally, rectally, or axillary.

🔑 The most commonly used site for taking the pulse is the wrist, called the radial pulse.

🔑 When taking the respirations of a resident, hold the wrist as if taking the pulse.

🔑 While measuring the blood pressure, you will be noting the systolic and diastolic pressure.

🔑 Always report any unusual vital signs to the nurse immediately.

🔑 Accuracy is very important when taking and recording vital signs.

Review Quiz Chapter 12
Vital Signs

Choose the best answer for the questions below.

1. Measuring the vital organs of the body is called taking

   (A) vital statistics.
   (B) vital signs.
   (C) blood pressure.
   (D) pulse.

2. Which of the following may cause the body temperature to increase?

   (A) Infection
   (B) Dehydration
   (C) Physical exercise
   (D) All of the above
   (E) A and B only

3. On glass mercury thermometers, each long line represents

   (A) one degree.
   (B) one number.
   (C) two tenths of a degree.
   (D) five tenths of a degree.

4. An oral temperature should *not* be used for the resident who

   (A) has dentures.
   (B) is a "mouth breather."
   (C) has received oral medications.
   (D) has eaten within the past hour.

5. The thermometer must be lubricated before

   (A) taking an axillary temperature.
   (B) taking a resident's temperature in the armpit.
   (C) taking the resident's temperature rectally.
   (D) placing the thermometer on the skin.

6. The rhythmic expansion and contraction of an artery is called

   (A) the rate.
   (B) the pulse.
   (C) the volume.
   (D) the blood pressure.

7. What body system are you checking when you measure pulse?

   (A) Respiration
   (B) Digestive
   (C) Circulatory
   (D) Elimination

8. The pulse felt at the wrist is the

   (A) carotid.
   (B) brachial.
   (C) apical.
   (D) radial.

9. Which of the following is *true* when counting the respirations of the resident?

   (A) Respirations are counted by watching the rise and fall of the chest
   (B) Counting of respirations is usually done when counting the pulse
   (C) The resident must be told when respirations are counted
   (D) All of the above
   (E) A and B only

10. Measurement of the amount of force exerted on the walls of the arteries as blood flows through is

    (A) pulse.
    (B) blood pressure.
    (C) pressure factor.
    (D) arterial pulse.

11. The resident's blood pressure reading is 130/84. The diastolic reading is

(A) 214
(B) 130
(C) 84
(D) 56

12. What is hypertension?

(A) High blood pressure
(B) Low blood pressure
(C) Nervousness
(D) Anxiety

13. What is your best action when you have taken the blood pressure of a resident and are not sure of the reading?

(A) Tell another nursing assistant to check it for you.
(B) Look up the last reading and record the same numbers.
(C) Tell the nurse about your uncertainty and ask her what to do.
(D) Forget the reading and try to take the resident's blood pressure the next day.

14. What should you do when the measurements of any vital sign are abnormally high or low?

(A) Record the measurements on the chart at the end of your shift.
(B) Alert the nurse immediately to the abnormal measurements.
(C) Tell the resident and ask what he or she would like you to do.
(D) Report to the nurse at the end of your work day.

15. The proper way to record the temperature, pulse, and respirations is to write the

(A) temperature first, pulse second, and respirations third.
(B) respirations first, pulse second, and temperature last.
(C) the temperature first, respirations second, and pulse third.
(D) Any order is acceptable.

16. You have just taken the vital signs of a resident. The readings were BP 132/82, T 98.8, P 74, R 32. Which, if any, of these readings were *not* in the normal range?

(A) Blood pressure
(B) Temperature
(C) Pulse
(D) Respirations
(E) None are normal

ANSWERS

1. B	6. B	11. C
2. D	7. C	12. A
3. A	8. D	13. C
4. B	9. E	14. B
5. C	10. B	15. A
		16. D

185

Appendix A

Test-Taking Methods and Guidelines

This appendix was written by Larry J. Bailey, Professor, Vocational Education Studies, Southern Illinois University, Carbondale, Illinois.

As you know, the Nursing Home Reform Act was passed by Congress in 1987. It says that all people working as nursing assistants before July 1, 1989 must satisfactorily complete a competency evaluation program. Those employed after July 1, 1989 must first enroll in a nursing assistant training program and then successfully complete a competency exam. The competency exam is made up of written questions and performances. In some cases, an oral exam may be given instead of a written exam.

The twelve chapters in this training manual are designed to give the information and skills needed to complete the competency exam. We want you to become eligible for, or to continue, working as a nursing assistant. *We want you to be successful.*

The material covered in Appendix A will help you prepare for the written portion of the competency exam. No one was born knowing how to take a test. Your performance on an exam can be improved by learning some test-taking methods and guidelines. By learning what to expect and by developing test-taking skills, you will know more and be more confident when taking the exam.

The Test

Unexpected surprises can make you tense and confused. Avoid this by learning as much as possible about a test in advance.

Standardized Tests

The exam you will be taking is **standardized.** This means that it was planned and written in such a way that everyone who takes the exam will be tested fairly. A test becomes standardized after it has been used, revised, and used again until it shows consistent results. The purpose is to establish an average score on the exam. The average score, called a **norm**, allows the results of one person's performance to be compared with those of many others across the country who have taken the same test.

A standardized test must be given in the same way. The test examiner must follow the same plan, read the same directions, and give only certain kinds of help. The situation at all test sites should be as much alike as possible. Scoring is standardized also. Every answer is scored according to definite rules.

Overview of the Test

The content of the **Nurse Aide Test** covers five main areas:

- Basic Nursing Skills (24)

- Basic Restorative Services (16)

- Mental Health and Social Service Needs (9)

- Personal Care Skills (13)

- Resident Rights (13)

The test is made up of 75 multiple-choice questions that are given in a 90-minute time period. The numbers in parentheses represent the approximate number of questions included for each area. Note that about one third of the test is devoted to Basic Nursing Skills.

The questions are not grouped by content area within the test booklet. Questions about Basic Nursing Skills, for instance, may appear anywhere throughout the test.

Answers to test questions are marked on the test booklet. A separate machine-readable information page is included to collect your name, sex, race, birthdate, education level, work experience, and state of residence.

Multiple-Choice Format

Most standardized tests use multiple-choice items. This is because multiple-choice questions can measure a variety of learning outcomes, from simple to complex. They also provide the most consistent results. The multiple-choice item consists of a **stem**, which presents a problem situation, and four or five possible choices called **alternatives**. The alternatives include the correct answer and several wrong answers called **distractors**. The stem may be a question or an incomplete statement, as shown.

- Question form:

  Q. Which of the following people is responsible for taking care of a resident ?

  Ⓐ Janitor
  Ⓑ Cook
  Ⓒ Nurse aide
  Ⓓ Dishwasher

- Incomplete-statement form:

Q. The care of a resident is the responsibility of a

    (A) janitor.
    (B) cook.
    (C) nurse aide.
    (D) dishwasher.

Although worded differently, both stems present the same problem. The alternatives in the examples contain only one correct answer. All distractors are clearly incorrect.

Another type of multiple-choice item is the **best-answer** form. In this form, the alternatives are all partially correct. But, one is clearly better than the others. Look at the example below.

- Best-answer form:

Q. Which of the following ethical behaviors is the MOST important?

    (A) Maintain a positive attitude.
    (B) Act as a responsible employee.
    (C) Be courteous to visitors.
    (D) Promote quality of life for each resident.

Other variations of the best-answer form may ask you "what is the FIRST thing to do," the "MOST helpful action," the "BEST response," or a similar kind of question. Whether the correct answer or best-answer form is used depends on the information given.

The examples use four alternatives. The chance of getting the correct answer by guessing is only one in four (25 percent).

Managing Test Anxiety

Test anxiety, or stress, is an emotional and physical response that the body makes to any demand made upon it. Stress may be good or bad. Its symptoms may be mild or severe. Mild stress may include feelings of anxiety, muscle tension, "butterflies" in the stomach, sweating, pounding of heart, dry mouth, and reduced ability to concentrate. You have probably had some of these feelings before.

Most stress, including test anxiety, doesn't last long. Once the stressful situation has passed, the symptoms disappear. You can learn to cope with test anxiety. The following guidelines will help you deal with test anxiety.

Understanding Stress

Two important characteristics to know about stress are that: (a) stress is normal and (b) stress can be good. If you are anxious about taking a test, you are not alone. Almost everyone has some test anxiety. The person who doesn't feel anxious about taking a test is usually the abnormal one.

You may be surprised to learn that stress can be good. Studies have shown that mild stress is associated with improved performance in athletes, entertainers, public speakers, and yes, test-takers. Butterflies, breathing faster, sweating, and other symptoms are automatic bodily responses to stressful situations. Stress can sharpen your attention, keep you alert, and give you greater energy.

Controlling Negative Thoughts

Factors that help cause test anxiety include negative thoughts and self-doubt. Perhaps you have thought such things as, "I am going to fail the exam," "I won't do well," or "What will my family and co-workers think when I don't pass." You must stop thinking such thoughts. Instead, say to yourself, "I have done this job successfully for many years. I know what it takes to be a nurse assistant. I am prepared to take this exam." Think of the exam as a chance to show what you know and can do. Positive thinking comes before positive action and positive results.

Preparing Yourself Physically

Learning information and guidelines help you prepare mentally for an exam. Physical preparation is also important. Some stressful situations cannot be predicted. An exam, however, is known in advance. During the time before the exam, try not to schedule other stressful activities. Eat well and get plenty of rest. Combine studying with exercise and relaxation. Don't stay up late cramming the night before an exam. This is the time for reviewing studied material and getting a good night's sleep.

If you feel stressful during the period before the exam, try this deep breathing method recommended by a stress management expert. Breathe deeply from your diaphragm. Do not move your chest and shoulders. You should feel your abdominal muscles expand as you breathe in and deflate when you breathe out. As you breathe out, your diaphragm and rib muscles relax, and your body may seem to sink down into the chair. Sixty seconds of deep breathing several times a day can help relieve stress.

Getting Ready for the Test_____

To prepare for a test, it is helpful to know whether it will contain **supply-type** or **selection-type** questions. Supply-type items are ones in which the test-taker supplies the answer. Essay and completion items are of this type. Selection-type items are ones in which the test-taker selects the answer from a number of possible answers.

True-false, multiple-choice, and matching items are of this type. The exam you will take is a selection-type exam because it is made up of only multiple-choice questions. You must select the correct answer from four different choices.

Studying for a selection-type test is done differently than for a supply-type test. In studying for an essay exam (supply-type), you should be ready to explain major theories, principles, or ideas; look for ways to compare and contrast concepts; list pros and cons for important issues; and provide definitions of basic terms.

Whereas the essay test tends to measure one's ability to organize, integrate, and express ideas, the multiple-choice test more often measures word-for-word memory. The same subject matter should be studied for selection-type items as for supply-type items. But, for selection-type items, concentrate on learning specific facts and information.

Multiple-choice questions are used in standardized tests, because they can be used to measure knowledge of facts and information as well as the application of facts and information. Knowledge items deal with such things as specific facts, common terms, methods and procedures, basic concepts and principles. Several examples of knowledge level items follow.

Q. The most basic human need is for

  Ⓐ food.
  Ⓑ oxygen.
  Ⓒ water.
  Ⓓ elimination.

Q. Which of the following is NOT a psychological need?

  Ⓐ Love
  Ⓑ Belong
  Ⓒ Exercise
  Ⓓ Identity

Application items measure a higher level of understanding. Here the test-taker must show that he or she not only understands the information but can also apply it to a situation. You must apply facts, concepts, principles, rules, methods, and theories to situations on the job. Following is an example of an application level question.

Q. The self-actualization needs of a resident can be assisted by

  Ⓐ listening to resident.
  Ⓑ calling resident by name.
  Ⓒ encouraging resident to be independent.
  Ⓓ praising accomplishments of resident.

You should be prepared to answer both knowledge and application level questions.

Studying and Reviewing

No matter what type of test you take, you must first learn the material. A good way to study for an exam is to use a system of index cards.

Obtain some 3 x 5 index cards or cut sheets of paper into a convenient size. On one side of the card write the name of terms, methods and procedures, basic concepts and principles, and other specific facts. On the reverse side of the card, write the answer, definition, explanation, or whatever else is important. Here are several examples.

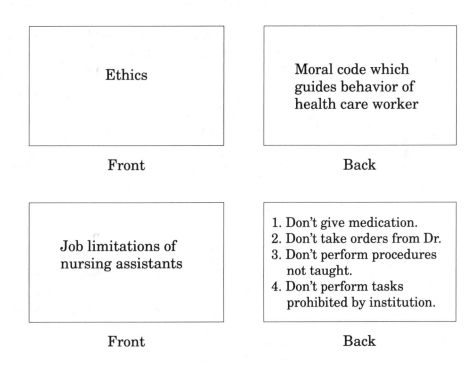

Ethics	Moral code which guides behavior of health care worker
Front	Back

Job limitations of nursing assistants	1. Don't give medication. 2. Don't take orders from Dr. 3. Don't perform procedures not taught. 4. Don't perform tasks prohibited by institution.
Front	Back

To study, look at the front of the card and try to remember what is written on the back. Turn the card over to see whether you are correct. After going through all the cards once, shuffle them and review the cards again. You want to be sure you know the information in any order.

As you review the cards, begin to sort them into two piles. One pile will be those you know well and the other pile will be those you are having trouble remembering. Once you have two piles, try to learn the more difficult information. Continue reviewing the cards until you are sure you have learned the material. Review the cards several times a day during the time before the exam.

There are a number of advantages to using this system. First, preparing the cards is a learning experience. Second, the cards are easy to carry with you in a pocket or purse. You can study them during spare moments throughout the day. Another advantage is that you can use the cards with a friend to quiz each other.

Taking the Practice Test

Practicing what is required to get ready for a test is excellent preparation for taking an actual exam. Taking a practice test can get you used to the kinds of directions that are given, the types of questions you will be expected to answer, and the process of marking machine-readable test booklets. It can also help you learn your strengths and weaknesses.

Appendix B contains a practice test that you will take. Treat the practice test as a real test. The practice test will be given under conditions as similar as possible to the real test.

Practice working with time limits. Note specifically the average time it takes you to complete a question. If you work at a steady pace, you should have plenty of time to complete the exam in 90 minutes.

After finishing the practice test, you will have an opportunity to score it and discuss specific questions. Use this opportunity to ask questions about questions that you missed. Use the results of the practice test to identify those areas you need to study. The score does not indicate whether you will pass or fail the competency test. Different states use different passing scores.

Taking the Test

To do well on a test, you should be at your best when you start. Eat a good breakfast (or lunch). Try to avoid anything that will make you tense. Leave for the test site early enough to arrive on time. Be sure to count for minor delays. Take a watch and two No. 2 black lead pencils with erasers. When you arrive, don't allow another person's last-minute questions or comments to disturb you. Follow these general rules for taking the test:

1. You will get verbal instructions before you take the test. You will complete an information page. Listen carefully to what the tester tells you to do. Remember that the tester is required to read or give very specific directions. The rules and directions are designed to treat fairly everyone who takes the test.

2. Before the test begins, take a few seconds to pay attention. Close your eyes and take several deep breaths. Remind yourself that you have studied well. Think positive.

3. Once you get the test and are told to begin, carefully read the directions. Look at any sample questions. Make sure that you understand how to mark answers on the test booklet or answer sheet. The test will probably be machine-scored, so be careful in recording answers.

4. You will have 90 minutes to answer 75 questions. This is a very generous amount of time. If you work at a steady pace you should have no problem finishing the test on time. Pause to check time and make sure that you are working at about the right speed. The examiner will post the time remaining.

5. Read the stem of the question and answer it in your own words without looking at the choices or alternatives. Then search for the alternative that matches your answer. Always read all of the alternatives. Answer "A" may be right, but answer "C" may be a better answer.

6. Some questions may ask you to analyze a situation or use what you have learned to solve a problem. If you don't know the answer immediately, it is often helpful to cross out unnecessary information. Distracting or extra information has been crossed out in the following example.

> Q.A resident who wears a wig ~~understands that the nurse aide will not talk about this information outside the facility because~~ this information is
>
> Ⓐ legal.
> Ⓑ confidential.
> Ⓒ negligent.
> Ⓓ cultural.

7. If you don't know an answer, circle the question and move on. You can come back to it later. This will save you time and help prevent the anxiety that comes from trying to remember. More importantly, you may find a clue to the answer somewhere in a later question.

8. If you encounter a very difficult question, don't worry. The rest of the test-takers will probably have trouble with it also. Keep in mind that a perfect score is not expected on a standardized test.

9. Be alert to such words as *not* and *except* that can completely change the intent of the question. Words in the stem are often *italicized*, CAPITALIZED, or are within "quotation marks" or (parentheses). Pay attention to such words. They are usually important to answering the question.

10. Standardized tests are revised several times so that the questions are clearly worded. So, do not read more into a question than is asked for. Do not look for trick questions or hidden meanings. If a question seems unclear, read it several times. Pay close attention to how it is worded. Try to relate the question to information and tasks with which you are familiar.

11. Avoid unfamiliar choices or alternatives. An alternative that you don't know, uses difficult words, seems complicated is probably incorrect.

12. If you don't know an answer, try to determine what the answer is not. Begin by crossing out alternatives that you know or feel are incorrect. If you can cross out two choices, you now have a 50% chance of choosing the correct answer of the remaining two alternatives.

13. Your score on the exam will be based on the number of questions answered correctly. So, be sure and answer all 75 items. There is no

penalty for guessing. This means that for those items that have you completely stumped, you should go ahead and guess. First, however, try to cross out choices that seem wrong.

14. As you near the end of the test, don't worry that some individuals may have finished already. Studies have shown that those who complete a test early do not necessarily get better scores than those who finish later.

15. When you get to the end of the test, go back and complete those items that you skipped earlier. You may now find that you remember the answer or are able to narrow down the answer.

16. If you complete all 75 questions and still have time remaining, review your answers. After rereading a question, you may have second thoughts about the answer. Should you change it? For those who have studied well for an exam, research shows that more of them are helped than hurt by changing answers. Don't change answers without a good reason. But, go ahead and change any answers that are based on new insights or recall of new information.

17. Before turning in the test, review how you marked the answers. Check to see that you answered every question, that you marked only one answer per question, that you marked the answer neatly and legibly, and that you completely erased any changes that were made. Erase any other marks you may have made on the test booklet.

After the Test

When time is called, you can breathe a sigh of relief. Listen carefully, however, to instructions about what to do with the test booklet. Information may also be given about when and how you will find out the results.

You will have to keep to yourself any questions you may have about some test questions. The examiner may not know or will not be allowed to give such information.

You may have to wait several weeks before you receive the test results. During this time, try not to worry. People tend to underestimate their performance on an exam. Thousands of people will take this exam. Be confident that you probably will score as well or better than most of them.

Appendix B
Practice Exam

Choose the best answer for the questions below.

1. The moral code that guides the behavior of the health care worker is called

   Ⓐ etiquette.
   Ⓑ ethics.
   Ⓒ care plan.
   Ⓓ dignity.

2. When communicating with the hearing-impaired resident, it is important to

   Ⓐ gently touch the resident to get attention.
   Ⓑ face the resident when talking.
   Ⓒ identify yourself to the resident.
   Ⓓ All of the above.

3. When you position a resident in side-lying position, you will use pillows to support

   Ⓐ the lower arm.
   Ⓑ the upper arm.
   Ⓒ the lower leg.
   Ⓓ the upper arm and leg.

4. Which of the following is a developmental task of the elderly resident?

   Ⓐ Increased social involvement
   Ⓑ Adjusting to losses
   Ⓒ Having a second career
   Ⓓ Adjusting to middle age

5. Which of the following would be considered an example of a pressure-relieving device?

   Ⓐ Quad cane
   Ⓑ Walker
   Ⓒ Sheepskin
   Ⓓ Pulley

6. Before replacing dentures into a resident's mouth,

   Ⓐ always wear gloves.
   Ⓑ allow resident to rinse mouth.
   Ⓒ store dentures in denture cup.
   Ⓓ floss the resident's teeth.

7. The electronic thermometer can be used for taking what kind of temperature?

   Ⓐ Oral temperatures only
   Ⓑ Oral and axillary
   Ⓒ Oral and rectal
   Ⓓ Oral, rectal, and axillary

8. When you have completed colostomy care for a resident, you will record any output as

   Ⓐ urinary output.
   Ⓑ a bowel movement.
   Ⓒ an emesis.
   Ⓓ homeostasis.

9. To properly give a bedbath,

   Ⓐ cover resident, and bathe entire body one part at a time.
   Ⓑ uncover resident, bathe entire body, then cover again.
   Ⓒ cover resident and bathe face, hands, underarms, back and genital area, one part at a time.
   Ⓓ cover resident, and take to shower in a shower chair.

10. When personal mail is sent to a long-term care facility, who has the right to open it first?

   Ⓐ Administrator
   Ⓑ Director of Nurses
   Ⓒ Resident
   Ⓓ State Inspectors

11. Mrs. Smith is an ambulatory resident. It would be most appropriate in a long-term care facility for her to have her lunch

   Ⓐ in her bed.
   Ⓑ in her room.
   Ⓒ in the dining room.
   Ⓓ at McDonald's.

12. Toenails of elderly residents should be trimmed

   Ⓐ before their tub bath.
   Ⓑ after their tub bath.
   Ⓒ during early A.M. care.
   Ⓓ only by a podiatrist.

13. When you are washing your hands, what part of the procedure removes the most germs?

   Ⓐ Using warm, running water
   Ⓑ Shaking water off your hands
   Ⓒ Using friction while washing your hands
   Ⓓ Drying hands thoroughly

14. Safety of the resident is the responsibility of the

   Ⓐ nurse in charge.
   Ⓑ nursing assistant.
   Ⓒ maintenance staff.
   Ⓓ All of the above

15. In order for a fire to occur, there must be a spark or flame, oxygen, and material that will burn. In most fire situations, where would the oxygen come from?

   Ⓐ The oxygen tanks
   Ⓑ The air itself
   Ⓒ The air conditioning
   Ⓓ The heating system

16. Why is it important to explain lifting procedures to residents before you're going to do them?

   Ⓐ To be polite
   Ⓑ To enlist their cooperation and help
   Ⓒ To prevent any arguments
   Ⓓ To provide communication

17. When removing soiled linen from the bed,

   Ⓐ shake linen gently to find lost items.
   Ⓑ roll it into a ball. Place on floor.
   Ⓒ place the linen into the hamper.
   Ⓓ All of the above.

18. A resident is waving one arm wildly, grabbing at throat area and coughing. Your best response is to

   Ⓐ get him a drink of water.
   Ⓑ give him oxygen immediately.
   Ⓒ allow him to continue coughing.
   Ⓓ slap his back four times firmly.

19. The charge nurse asks you to check vital signs on Mrs. Jones. You will check her

   Ⓐ blood pressure and pulse.
   Ⓑ temperature and pulse.
   Ⓒ temperature, pulse, and respirations.
   Ⓓ blood pressure, temperature, pulse, and respirations.

20. When a resident with a paralyzed side wants to brush his own teeth, you should

   (A) brush his teeth for him anyway.
   (B) set out the supplies and allow him to do it.
   (C) explain you are happy to help him and do it for him.
   (D) guide his toothbrush through the procedure.

21. Decubitus ulcers are

   (A) prevented by good skin care.
   (B) caused by pressure.
   (C) called bedsores.
   (D) All of the above

22. One of your residents states, "I think the batteries are dead in my hearing aid—can't hear a thing!" How can you tell if the battery is working or not?

   (A) Remove hearing aid, turn up volume, and listen for whistling.
   (B) Remove hearing aid, take battery out and inspect it for leakage.
   (C) Explain to the resident that the battery can only be checked with a battery tester.
   (D) Notify the hearing aid company to call on the resident.

23. The correct positioning of the resident's body is called

   (A) muscle development.
   (B) body mechanics.
   (C) body alignment.
   (D) adaptive positioning.

24. What kind of problems exist for a resident who needs elastic stockings (TED sox)?

   (A) Musculoskeletal
   (B) Respiratory
   (C) Circulatory
   (D) Digestive

25. The nurse tells you to ambulate Mrs. Black in Room 202. This means to

   (A) sit her in the wheelchair.
   (B) sit her on the edge of the bed.
   (C) walk her to the bathroom.
   (D) walk her up and down the hall.

26. To properly wash the eyes while giving a bedbath, you would

   (A) wipe from outer side of eye to inner side.
   (B) wipe from inner side of eye to outer side.
   (C) start at middle of eye, then side to side.
   (D) never wipe the eye, use eye drops.

27. An example of meeting the psychological needs of a resident would be to assist with

   (A) eating supper.
   (B) going to sleep.
   (C) saying prayers.
   (D) getting dressed.

28. Microorganisms are completely destroyed by

   (A) sterilization.
   (B) hand washing.
   (C) disinfection.
   (D) medical asepsis.

29. When you find a resident who appears to have fallen on the floor, your first action is

   (A) run to get help.
   (B) put the resident in bed.
   (C) stay with the resident.
   (D) call the paramedics.

30. The skin of the elderly resident becomes

   (A) thicker.
   (B) fatter.
   (C) thinner.
   (D) brittle.

31. Standard equipment in the resident's "unit" is the

    Ⓐ TV, electric bed, and telephone.
    Ⓑ wheelchair, stretcher, and mechanical lift.
    Ⓒ hopper, sink, table, and work counter.
    Ⓓ bedside stand, bed, chair, and over-bed table

32. Your resident's care plan states to check BP q.i.d. This means to check

    Ⓐ bladder pressure every day.
    Ⓑ blood pressure four times a day.
    Ⓒ blood pressure every other day.
    Ⓓ bladder pressure four times a day.

33. You have taken a resident's rectal temperature and the thermometer reads 100 degrees. From your knowledge about body temperature, the oral temperature on this resident is

    Ⓐ 101.
    Ⓑ 99.
    Ⓒ 98.
    Ⓓ 97.

34. Mrs. Green is a 70-year-old resident who has been on bedrest with pneumonia for three days. You note a reddened area on her back. Your response is to

    Ⓐ encourage her to get up and move about.
    Ⓑ apply a dressing to the area.
    Ⓒ apply a heating pad to the area.
    Ⓓ report the area to the nurse.

35. If you are assisting a resident with ADLs, you are helping with

    Ⓐ activities of daily living.
    Ⓑ activities during leisure.
    Ⓒ proper alignment.
    Ⓓ A.M. care.

36. When residents are helpless and lay in one position for too long a period of time, there is risk of developing

    Ⓐ contractures.
    Ⓑ atrophy.
    Ⓒ bedsores.
    Ⓓ All of the above

37. When you take a resident's pulse, you are using a(an)

    Ⓐ artery.
    Ⓑ vein.
    Ⓒ capillary.
    Ⓓ All of the above

38. After completing the care for a resident who required isolation procedures, what is your *first* step in removing your gown, gloves, and mask?

    Ⓐ Remove mask, touching only ties.
    Ⓑ Untie waist ties and tie in front of gown.
    Ⓒ Untie neck ties and loosen gown at shoulders.
    Ⓓ Grasp cuff of glove and pull off.

39. The strongest muscles you should use for lifting are in your

    Ⓐ buttocks.
    Ⓑ thighs.
    Ⓒ back.
    Ⓓ abdomen.

40. Restraints require a doctor's order and must be released every

    Ⓐ half-hour.
    Ⓑ hour.
    Ⓒ two hours.
    Ⓓ four hours.

41. When residents are admitted to a long-term care facility, they

    (A) no longer have the right to vote.
    (B) can continue to vote in elections.
    (C) need permission to leave the facility.
    (D) cannot drive a car.

42. Exposing a resident unnecessarily would be a threat to the right to

    (A) privacy.
    (B) security.
    (C) acceptance.
    (D) belonging.

43. Basic human needs are

    (A) different for each person.
    (B) varied in men and women.
    (C) the same for all people.
    (D) different, depending on age.

44. When a resident has a need for recognition, you can easily provide this by

    (A) calling the resident by name.
    (B) explaining procedures.
    (C) providing privacy.
    (D) turning on the TV.

45. A resident who frequently wanders at night, becomes easily agitated and cannot be calmed down, is displaying symptoms of

    (A) mental retardation.
    (B) multiple sclerosis.
    (C) Alzheimer's.
    (D) delusions.

46. When you give a bedbath, you always obtain clean bath water after washing the

    (A) genital area.
    (B) legs and feet.
    (C) armpits.
    (D) navel area.

47. An example of an adaptive device to help a resident in dressing and grooming tasks would be a

    (A) handroll.
    (B) transfer belt.
    (C) long-handled shoe horn.
    (D) four-pronged cane.

48. Mr. Brown's TPR is 96.8-104-30. Which, if any, are normal?

    (A) Temperature
    (B) Pulse
    (C) Respirations
    (D) None are normal
    (E) All are normal

49. Who is responsible to check the scale for balance before taking a resident's weight?

    (A) Charge nurse
    (B) Nursing assistant
    (C) Maintenance staff
    (D) Administrator

50. An occupied bed is made with the

    (A) resident in a chair.
    (B) assistance of the nurse.
    (C) resident in the bed.
    (D) assistance of the resident.

51. Identify the six essential nutrients for good nutrition.

    (A) Carbohydrates, proteins, vitamins, minerals, amino acids, and water.
    (B) Carbohydrates, proteins, fats, vitamins, minerals, and water.
    (C) Proteins, fats, vitamins, minerals, calcium, and water.
    (D) Carbohydrates, proteins, fats, vitamins, calcium, and iron.

52. The term edema means

    (A) abnormal swelling in the tissues.
    (B) loss of fluid from the tissues.
    (C) instilling fluid into the rectum.
    (D) the same as dehydration.

53. When counting a resident's pulse, you notice it is weak and irregular. Proper technique would be to count

   Ⓐ for one full minute and record.
   Ⓑ for 30 seconds, double number, and record.
   Ⓒ for 15 seconds, multiply by 4, and record.
   Ⓓ the pulse in two separate locations.

54. One of your residents wants to see the chaplain immediately, but the chaplain has left for the day. What should you do?

   Ⓐ Ignore the request. The chaplain will be back tomorrow.
   Ⓑ Tell the resident the chaplain has left for the day.
   Ⓒ Ask the resident, "Why do you want to see him?"
   Ⓓ Refer the request to the nurse in charge.

55. The charge nurse reports to you that Mrs. White has high blood pressure. Another word for this is

   Ⓐ hypotension.
   Ⓑ systolic.
   Ⓒ hypertension.
   Ⓓ diastolic.

56. When you "log roll" a resident, before placing on a bedpan, place your hands on the resident's

   Ⓐ shoulder and hip.
   Ⓑ waist and hip.
   Ⓒ hip and legs.
   Ⓓ arm and leg.

57. When you take a resident's blood pressure, you are measuring

   Ⓐ the volume of blood.
   Ⓑ the force of the heart.
   Ⓒ how fast the heart is beating.
   Ⓓ the rhythm of the pulse.

58. It is important for the nursing assistant to know that the skin of the geriatric resident produces

   Ⓐ more oil.
   Ⓑ less oil.
   Ⓒ no oil.

59. When a resident has an ongoing like or dislike for certain foods, it may be because of

   Ⓐ the surroundings in which it is served.
   Ⓑ your influence on the resident.
   Ⓒ family customs, cultural influence.
   Ⓓ a decrease in appetite.

60. You have inflated the blood pressure cuff to 160 mm. As you release the air, you immediately hear the sound of the heart. What should you do next?

   Ⓐ Continue to inflate the cuff until the sound is gone.
   Ⓑ Record the sound as the diastolic pressure.
   Ⓒ Deflate the cuff entirely and reinflate to a higher number.
   Ⓓ Loosen the cuff slowly.

61. During Mrs. Smith's bath, you observe that her face is very flushed and her skin feels warm to the touch. The best way to report this to the team leader is

   Ⓐ "Mrs. Smith has a fever."
   Ⓑ "I think Mrs. Smith is getting sick."
   Ⓒ "You should take Mrs. Smith's temperature."
   Ⓓ "Mrs. Smith's face is flushed and her skin fells warm."

62. Effective communication is a very important part of your job as a nursing assistant. When you smile at a resident, what kind of communication are you using?

   Ⓐ Sign language
   Ⓑ Body language
   Ⓒ Oral communication
   Ⓓ Verbal communication

63. "STAT" means

 (A) as desired.
 (B) as necessary.
 (C) at once.
 (D) at mealtime.

64. When a resident is on I&O, you will do your recording as

 (A) ounces.
 (B) cups.
 (C) cubic centimeters.
 (D) centigrade.

65. When you sit a resident up on the edge of the bed and the resident becomes dizzy, your best action is to

 (A) sit the resident in the chair.
 (B) lay the resident down and call the nurse.
 (C) tell the resident it will be okay in a few minutes.
 (D) put the resident into a wheelchair and take to the nurse.

66. The extent a person is capable of moving a joint is called

 (A) flexibility.
 (B) contractures.
 (C) restoration.
 (D) range of motion.

67. When a resident has died and you are doing postmortem care, the right to privacy is

 (A) no longer necessary.
 (B) still protected after death.
 (C) only for the family.
 (D) All of the above

68. When you assist the resident to get ready for mealtime, you would also include checking their

 (A) weight.
 (B) blood pressure.
 (C) need to use the toilet.
 (D) need to say grace.

69. If a resident leaves 1/4 of an 8 ounce glass of milk on the tray, how much would you record as taken?

 (A) 60 cc.
 (B) 120 cc.
 (C) 180 cc.
 (D) 240cc.

70. Mrs. Smith's blood pressure is 142/88. You will record the systolic reading as

 (A) 230.
 (B) 142.
 (C) 88.
 (D) 54.

71. Mr. Jones, a bedridden patient, states he has to move his bowels. You would help him use the

 (A) bedpan.
 (B) urinal.
 (C) urinary bag.
 (D) colostomy bag

72. When you communicate to residents in a therapeutic manner called, "therapeutic communication," what are you specifically doing?

 (A) Preparing them for a visit from their doctor.
 (B) Healing or improving an existing situation.
 (C) Planning to take them to physical therapy.
 (D) Encouraging them to get involved in activities.

73. Helping residents reach their highest level of ability is the goal of

 (A) range of motion.
 (B) disease prevention.
 (C) rehabilitation.
 (D) contractures.

74. A good ethical practice as a nursing assistant would be to

Ⓐ share your problems with the resident.
Ⓑ use care with the resident's belongings.
Ⓒ discuss the resident's condition at break.
Ⓓ borrow items from the resident's dresser.

75. To properly practice what you have been taught about universal precautions, it is best to

Ⓐ always wear a mask.
Ⓑ dispose of trash first.
Ⓒ scrub your hands with a brush.
Ⓓ carry gloves at all times.

Appendix C
Procedure Review

Procedure 1
Postmortem Care

Name _____

Social Security Number _____

Certification Number _____

	DATE S/U	DATE S/U	DATE S/U
1. Wash your hands			
2. Gather supplies: shroud kit with gown and identification tags, basin of warm water, washcloth, towels, and gloves.			
3. Give privacy.			
4. Treat the body with respect.			
5. Wear gloves.			
6. Close the eyes by gently pulling eyelids down over eyes.			
7. Place cleaned dentures in mouth.			
8. Close the mouth. A rolled up washcloth may be placed under chin to keep jaw closed.			
9. Remove all tubing from body.			
10. Bathe the body, comb hair, and straighten arms and legs.			
11. Apply clean dressings to wounds, if necessary.			
12. Pad the genital area.			
13. Put shroud or gown on body.			
14. Attach identification tag to body as indicated by facility policy.			
15. Replace any soiled linen.			
16. Tidy area of unit.			

DATE SATISFACTORY DEMONSTRATION

INSTRUCTOR INITIALS

TOTAL HOURS FOR THIS CANDIDATE TO COMPLETE PROCEDURE

LOCATION

COMMENTS

(continued next page

	DATE S/U	DATE S/U	DATE S/U
17. Collect all belongings, place them in bag, and label them correctly. Usually these are given to the resident's family.			
18. Give privacy to the family when they visit the body.			
19. Follow facility policy, if necessary, to bring body to morgue.			
20. Clean unit as directed after body has been removed.			

Procedure 2

Hand Washing

Name _____

Social Security Number _____

Certification Number _____

	DATE S/U	DATE S/U	DATE S/U
1. Stand away from sink. Uniform and hands must not touch sink.			
2. Turn on water, using a paper towel, adjust water to warm, comfortable temperature.			
3. Wet hands and wrists.			
4. Apply soap over hands and wrists working into a lather.			
5. Use friction when washing hands, fingers, and wrists.			
6. Wash for one minute.			
7. Rinse hands and wrists under running water.			
8. Do not shake water from hands.			
9. Dry hands and wrists with clean paper towel.			
10. Turn off faucets, using clean paper towel.			
11. Throw away paper towel.			

DATE SATISFACTORY DEMONSTRATION

INSTRUCTOR INITIALS

TOTAL HOURS FOR THIS CANDIDATE TO COMPLETE PROCEDURE

LOCATION

COMMENTS

Procedure **3**

Isolation Procedures

Name _____

Social Security Number _____

Certification Number _____

	DATE S/U	DATE S/U	DATE S/U
A. Procedure for gowning, gloving, and masking using disposable gown, gloves, and mask			
1. Remove your jewelry.			
2. Wash your hands and dry them thoroughly.			
3. Put on mask, adjust over nose and mouth, and tie securely at back of head.			
4. Put on gown, making certain gown overlaps in back covering all clothing.			
5. Tie neck ties.			
6. Tie waist ties, making certain gown is overlapping.			
7. Put on gloves covering cuff of gown with top edge of glove.			
B. Procedure for removal			
1. Make sure that all jobs in isolation unit are completed and that the resident is comfortable and safe.			
2. Untie waist ties and tie in front of gown. This prevents contaminated ties from touching your uniform.			
3. Remove first glove by grasping cuff of glove and pulling off. Throw away in trash container.			
4. Remove second glove by placing bare hand inside the cuff of glove and pulling it off. Throw away in trash container.			
5. Grasp the neck ties of the gown and untie. The neck ties are considered a clean area.			

DATE
SATISFACTORY
DEMONSTRATION

INSTRUCTOR
INITIALS

TOTAL HOURS FOR
THIS CANDIDATE
TO COMPLETE
PROCEDURE

LOCATION

COMMENTS

(continued next page)

	DATE S/U	DATE S/U	DATE S/U
6. Loosen the gown at the shoulders, touching only the inside of the gown.			
7. Slip fingers of one hand under cuff of gown at opposite arm. Do not touch outside of gown. Pull it down over hand.			
8. With hand inside of gown, pull gown off of other arm.			
9. Fold and roll gown with the contaminated side in.			
10. Throw away in trash container.			
11. Remove mask by grasping only the ties.			
12. Throw away mask in trash container.			
13. Use paper towel to turn on faucets.			
14. Wash hands.			
15. Open door with paper towel.			
16. Repeat hand washing or use disinfectant as policy of your facility indicates.			

Procedure 4

Applying a Vest Restraint

Name _____

Social Security Number _____

Certification Number _____

	DATE S/U	DATE S/U	DATE S/U	
1. Wash your hands.				**DATE SATISFACTORY DEMONSTRATION**
2. Explain to resident who you are and what you are going to do.				
3. Get help, if necessary.				
4. Get a vest restraint.				
5. Give privacy.				**INSTRUCTOR INITIALS**
6. Slip the resident's arms through the armholes of the vest.				
7. Make sure clothing under restraint is not wrinkled and vest fits smoothly.				
8. Fasten ties or secure vest to fit comfortably but not tightly.				
9. Bring the straps through the slots at sides of vest.				**TOTAL HOURS FOR THIS CANDIDATE TO COMPLETE PROCEDURE**
10. Tie the straps of the vest to the bed frame or in the back of chair or wheelchair.				
11. Use knot recommended by facility policy.				
12. Place call light within resident's reach.				
13. Leave resident comfortable and safe.				
14. Wash your hands.				**LOCATION**
15. According to policy, record or report the resident's skin condition and reaction to restraint application.				**COMMENTS**

Procedure 5

Making the Unoccupied Bed

Name _____

Social Security Number _____

Certification Number _____

	DATE S/U	DATE S/U	DATE S/U
1. Wash your hands.			
2. Introduce yourself to the resident.			
3. Explain to resident what you are going to do.			
4. Gather supplies needed: two large sheets, linen draw sheet, plastic or rubber draw sheet, pillow case, laundry bag or hamper, and clean bedspread, if needed.			
5. Carry linens away from your uniform.			
6. Place linens on clean area near bed in order of use. From bottom to top: pillow case, spread, sheet, linen draw sheet, plastic draw sheet, and sheets.			
7. Place bed in high, flat position.			
8. Remove and fold spread if you are reusing it.			
9. Remove soiled linens by rolling them into a ball without touching your uniform.			
10. Place soiled linens in laundry bag.			
11. Place bottom sheet on bed, centering the lengthwise middle fold of sheet in middle of bed.			
12. Open sheet.			
13. Place sheet with small hem even with foot edge of mattress.			
14. Tuck top of sheet under top of mattress.			
15. Miter corner of sheet at head of bed. Secure upper and lower corners of fitted sheet.			
16. Tuck in bottom sheet on side of bed, working from head to foot.			

DATE SATISFACTORY DEMONSTRATION

INSTRUCTOR INITIALS

TOTAL HOURS FOR THIS CANDIDATE TO COMPLETE PROCEDURE

LOCATION

COMMENTS

(continued next page)

	DATE S/U	DATE S/U	DATE S/U
17. Place plastic draw sheet over middle one third of bed.			
18. Tuck edge of plastic sheet under mattress.			
19. Place linen draw sheet over plastic sheet, covering entire plastic sheet.			
20. Tuck linen draw sheet under mattress.			
21. Place top sheet on bed, centering the lengthwise middle fold in center of bed.			
22. Position sheet with top edge even with top of mattress.			
23. Tuck bottom of sheet under mattress at foot of bed.			
24. Place bedspread on bed.			
25. Position bedspread about four inches above top edge of mattress.			
26. Miter top linens at foot of bed.			
27. Move to other side of bed.			
28. Pull and smooth out bottom sheet.			
29. Tuck bottom sheet under mattress at head of bed pulling tight.			
30. Miter corner of sheet at head of bed. Secure upper and lower corners of fitted sheet.			
31. Pull and tightly tuck side of bottom sheet under mattress.			
32. Pull plastic sheet tightly.			
33. Tuck plastic sheet under mattress, pulling and tucking from middle of plastic sheet first. Then pull and tuck edges of sheet.			
34. Pull linen draw sheet tightly.			
35. Tuck linen draw sheet under mattress, pulling and tucking from middle of draw sheet first. Then pull and tuck edges.			
36. Check foundation of bed. Make sure bed is smooth and wrinkle free.			
37. Pull and smooth top sheet.			

(continued next page)

	DATE S/U	DATE S/U	DATE S/U
38. Pull and smooth spread.			
39. Tuck sheet and spread under foot of mattress.			
40. Miter top linens at foot of bed.			
41. Fold spread back about 30 inches.			
42. Make cuff on top sheet by folding back about four inches at top edge of sheet.			
43. Place pillow on bed.			
44. Insert zippered end of pillow in pillowcase toward closed end of pillowcase.			
45. Straighten pillowcase on pillow			
46. Place pillow at head of bed.			
47. Cover pillow with bedspread.			
48. Place bed in low position.			
49. Place call light within resident's reach.			
50. Assure resident's comfort and safety.			
51. Wash your hands.			

Procedure 6

Clearing an Obstructed Airway (Heimlich Maneuver)

Name _____

Social Security Number _____

Certification Number _____

	DATE S/U	DATE S/U	DATE S/U	
Clearing an Obstructed Airway in a Conscious Adult:				**DATE SATISFACTORY DEMONSTRATION**
1. Call for the nurse immediately.				
2. If resident is sitting or standing, stand behind him.				
3. Wrap your arms around his waist.				
4. Make a fist with one hand.				**INSTRUCTOR INITIALS**
5. Place the thumb of your fist against the resident's abdomen, just above the navel and below the tip of the breastbone.				
6. Grasp fist with other hand.				
7. Push in and upward on abdomen with a quick thrust.				
8. Repeat until the foreign body comes out or resident loses consciousness. Proceed to CPR only if you've had instruction. Otherwise, call nurse.				**TOTAL HOURS FOR THIS CANDIDATE TO COMPLETE PROCEDURE**
Clearing an Obstructed Airway in an Unconscious Adult				
It is extremely important that you know of your facility's policy regarding this procedure. Often this is the responsibility of the nurse. The procedure is listed here for your general understanding only.				
1. Call for help, but do not leave.				**LOCATION**
2. Lower resident to the floor and position him on his back				
3. Open airway by tilting head back and lifting jaw.				**COMMENTS**
4. Use finger sweep to try to clear foreign object from mouth. Do not push it further down throat.				

(continued next page)

	DATE S/U	DATE S/U	DATE S/U
5. Try to give two breaths.			
6. Straddle victim.			
7. Place heel of hand above navel. Thrust 6 to 10 times.			
8. Try to give two breaths.			
9. Repeat thrusts, sweeping mouth, and giving breaths until object is dislodged.			
10. Continue until airway is open, help arrives, or rescuer cannot continue.			

Procedure 7

Positioning the Resident in Supine Position

Name _____

Social Security Number _____

Certification Number _____

	DATE S/U	DATE S/U	DATE S/U	
1. Wash your hands.				DATE SATISFACTORY DEMONSTRATION
2. Explain to resident who you are and what you are going to do.				
3. Give privacy.				
4. Lock bed wheels.				
5. Raise bed to comfortable working level.				
6. Lower side rail on working side after positioning bed.				INSTRUCTOR INITIALS
7. Position resident, lying on his back.				
8. Place resident's arms at sides in comfortable, functional position, supporting with pillows, if necessary.				
9. Check for good body alignment.				
10. Pad bony prominences of elbows and heels, if indicated.				TOTAL HOURS FOR THIS CANDIDATE TO COMPLETE PROCEDURE
11. Leave resident comfortable.				
12. Raise side rails.				
13. Position call light within resident's reach.				
14. Place bed in low position.				
15. Wash your hands.				LOCATION
16. Report to nurse or record any skin irritation or redness.				COMMENTS

Procedure 8

Positioning a Resident in a Side-Lying Position

Name _____

Social Security Number _____

Certification Number _____

	DATE S/U	DATE S/U	DATE S/U
1. Wash your hands.			
2. Explain to resident who you are and what you are going to do.			
3. Gather supplies.			
4. Give privacy.			
5. Lock bed wheels.			
6. Raise bed to comfortable working level.			
7. Lower side rail on working side after positioning bed.			
8. Begin this procedure by standing on the side opposite from which the resident will lie.			
9. Use proper body mechanics to move resident.			
10. Place one of your arms under resident's shoulder. Place other arm under resident's back.			
11. Move upper part of resident's body towards you.			
12. Place one of your arms under resident's waist and other arm under resident's thighs.			
13. Move resident's midsection toward you.			
14. Move resident's legs toward you.			
15. Raise side rail.			
16. Go to other side of bed. Lower side rail.			
17. Flex and place resident's arm nearest you and toward head of bed. Place resident's other arm across chest.			

DATE SATISFACTORY DEMONSTRATION

INSTRUCTOR INITIALS

TOTAL HOURS FOR THIS CANDIDATE TO COMPLETE PROCEDURE

LOCATION

COMMENTS

(continued next page)

	DATE S/U	DATE S/U	DATE S/U
18. Cross resident's leg farthest from you across nearest leg.			
19. Place one of your hands on resident's shoulder. Place the other hand on hip.			
20. Roll resident toward you.			
21. Adjust pillow under resident's head.			
22. Flex and place upper arm on pillow.			
23. Place hand in functional position.			
24. Flex and place upper leg on pillow. Upper leg and pillow should not rest on lower leg.			
25. Raise side rail. Go to other side of bed.			
26. Lower side rail.			
27. Position pillow alongside resident's back.			
28. Raise side rail.			
29. Check for good alignment.			
30. Pad bony prominences of elbows and heels, if indicated.			
31. Leave resident comfortable.			
32. Raise side rails.			
33. Position call light within resident's reach.			
34. Place bed in low position.			
35. Wash your hands.			
36. Report to nurse or record any skin irritation or redness.			

Procedure 9

Moving a Resident Up in Bed

Name _____

Social Security Number _____

Certification Number _____

	DATE S/U	DATE S/U	DATE S/U
1. Wash your hands.			
2. Introduce yourself to resident.			
3. Explain to resident what you are going to do. Use good body mechanics throughout this procedure.			
4. Provide privacy.			
5. Lock bed wheels.			
6. Raise bed to comfortable working level.			
7. Lower head of bed.			
8. Remove pillow from under resident's head.			
9. Lean pillow against headboard.			
10. Stand next to bed.			
11. Ask resident to bend knees and put feet flat on mattress.			
12. If resident is able, ask him to bend arms at sides. Place hands on bed. Push with hands when told to do so.			
13. Slide one hand and arm under resident's upper back and shoulders.			
14. Slide other arm under resident's hips and buttocks.			
15. Instruct resident to push with hands and feet on count of three.			
16. On count of three, move resident to head of bed.			
17. Replace pillow under head.			
18. Check to see if resident is in good alignment.			

DATE SATISFACTORY DEMONSTRATION

INSTRUCTOR INITIALS

TOTAL HOURS FOR THIS CANDIDATE TO COMPLETE PROCEDURE

LOCATION

COMMENTS

(continued next page)

	DATE S/U	DATE S/U	DATE S/U
19. Raise side rail and lower bed.			
20. Leave resident comfortable and safe with call light within reach.			
21. Tidy area.			
22. Wash your hands.			
23. Record or report resident's tolerance to procedure and skin condition.			

Procedure 10

Ambulating the Resident with a Walker or Cane

Name _____

Social Security Number _____

Certification Number _____

	DATE S/U	DATE S/U	DATE S/U
1. Wash your hands.			
2. Explain to resident who you are and what you are going to do. Use good body mechanics throughout this procedure.			
3. Gather supplies: cane or walker, transfer belt, resident's robe, and shoes, if necessary.			
4. Give privacy.			
5. Lock bed wheels.			
6. Check cane or walker for safety.			
7. If resident is in bed, lower side rail.			
8. Raise head of bed.			
9. Help resident sit on edge of bed by supporting shoulders while resident swings legs across and off side of bed.			
10. Help resident into robe and shoes.			
11. Put transfer belt around resident's waist, fitting closely and securely.			
12. Put cane in resident's hand or walker in front of resident.			
13. Help resident stand. Grasp the transfer belt underhand at resident's side.			
14. When resident is standing and is balanced, ask him if he is dizzy or weak.			
15. Walk beside resident. Hold transfer belt at resident's back.			

DATE SATISFACTORY DEMONSTRATION

INSTRUCTOR INITIALS

TOTAL HOURS FOR THIS CANDIDATE TO COMPLETE PROCEDURE

LOCATION

COMMENTS

(continued next page)

	DATE S/U	DATE S/U	DATE S/U
16. Walk distance recommended by care plan or nurse's instruction.			
17. Encourage resident to walk with back straight and head up.			
18. Help the resident to a chair or bed.			
19. Remove transfer belt. Remove robe and shoes, if resident is returning to bed.			
20. Raise side rails, if resident is returned to bed.			
21. Leave resident comfortable and safe with call light within reach.			
22. Replace equipment, and tidy area.			
23. Wash your hands.			
24. Record or report distance walked and resident's tolerance.			

Procedure 11

Transferring a Resident from Bed to Wheelchair

Name _____

Social Security Number _____

Certification Number _____

	DATE S/U	DATE S/U	DATE S/U
1. Wash your hands.			
2. Explain to resident who you are and what you are going to do. Use good body mechanics throughout this procedure.			
3. Gather supplies: wheelchair, transfer belt, resident's robe, shoes or slippers, and covering for lap.			
4. Give privacy.			
5. Position wheelchair so resident's stronger side will be closest to wheelchair when resident is sitting on edge of bed. Place wheelchair within one foot of bed at slight angle.			
6. Raise or remove foot rests. Lock wheelchair brakes.			
7. Raise head of bed.			
8. Lock bed brakes. Lower side rail.			
9. Put on resident's shoes or slippers.			
10. Cross weaker leg over stronger leg.			
11. Help resident sit on edge of bed.			
12. Check whether resident seems weak.			
13. Help resident put on robe.			
14. Put transfer belt securely around resident's waist.			
15. Use transfer belt to move resident to edge of bed until resident's feet are flat on floor.			
16. Grasp transfer belt at resident's waist with both hands, using an underhand grasp.			

DATE SATISFACTORY DEMONSTRATION

INSTRUCTOR INITIALS

TOTAL HOURS FOR THIS CANDIDATE TO COMPLETE PROCEDURE

LOCATION

COMMENTS

(continued next page)

	DATE S/U	DATE S/U	DATE S/U
17. Support resident's weaker side.			
18. Tell resident to push off bed with his stronger hand after counting to three.			
19. Help resident stand.			
20. Turn resident to wheelchair toward his stronger side. Keep a good grasp on transfer belt with both hands.			
21. Be sure that resident can feel edge of wheelchair seat before he sits.			
22. Tell resident to place stronger hand on wheelchair arm. Sit resident in chair.			
23. Remove transfer belt.			
24. Put wheelchair safety belt on the resident.			
25. Adjust wheelchair leg rests and footrests.			
26. Place resident's feet on footrests.			
27. Cover lap with covering.			
28. Leave resident comfortable and safe with call light within reach.			
29. Replace equipment. Tidy area.			
30. Wash your hands.			
31. Record or report resident's tolerance and ability.			

Procedure 12

Transferring a Resident from Wheelchair to Toilet

Name _____

Social Security Number _____

Certification Number _____

	DATE S/U	DATE S/U	DATE S/U
1. Wash your hands.			
2. Explain to resident who you are and what you are going to do. Use good body mechanics throughout this procedure.			
3. Give privacy.			
4. Make sure bathroom is empty.			
5. Bring resident in wheelchair to bathroom.			
6. Close bathroom door.			
7. Position wheelchair at right angle to toilet. That is, the side of the wheelchair faces the front of the toilet.			
8. Release wheelchair security belt.			
9. Fasten transfer belt around resident's waist, if required.			
10. Lock wheelchair brakes.			
11. Tell resident to push up from wheelchair while you lift him with transfer belt. Count to three to match movements.			
12. Ask resident to hold bathroom grab bar.			
13. Help resident stand, giving him time to get balanced.			
14. Turn resident so he is standing in front of toilet.			
15. Lower resident's underwear.			
16. Help resident sit on toilet.			
17. Be sure call light is close to resident.			

DATE SATISFACTORY DEMONSTRATION

INSTRUCTOR INITIALS

TOTAL HOURS FOR THIS CANDIDATE TO COMPLETE PROCEDURE

LOCATION

COMMENTS

(continued next page)

	DATE S/U	DATE S/U	DATE S/U
18. Give privacy.			
19. Return when resident says he is done.			
20. Put on gloves to help the resident wipe excess bowel movement or urine.			
21. To help him stand, ask resident to hold onto bathroom grab bar and pull himself up. Match movements on the count of three. Grasp onto transfer belt at resident's waist.			
22. Pull underwear up.			
23. Smooth the resident's clothing.			
24. Turn and seat resident into locked wheelchair.			
25. Help resident wash hands.			
26. Remove resident from bathroom.			
27. Take off transfer belt.			
28. Take resident where he wants to go.			
29. Place call light within resident's reach.			
30. Leave resident comfortable and safe.			
31. Tidy area.			
32. Wash your hands.			
33. Record or report resident's tolerance to procedure and any unusual urine or stool.			

Procedure 13

Giving Passive Range-of-Motion Exercises

Name _____

Social Security Number _____

Certification Number _____

	DATE S/U	DATE S/U	DATE S/U
1. Explain to resident who you are and what you are going to do.			
2. Use good body mechanics throughout this procedure.			
3. Wash your hands.			
4. Give privacy.			
5. Raise bed to comfortable working height.			
6. Lower side rail on working side.			
7. Position resident in supine position.			
8. Exercise the extremities as indicated on care plan, supporting the limbs at closest joints.			
A. Head and neck:			
1. Lean head forward, bringing chin to chest.			
2. Lean head backward with chin up.			
3. Turn head from side to side.			
4. Turn head back and forth in a circular motion.			
B. Shoulders, arms, and elbows:			
1. Move arm over head, with arm touching top of head.			
2. Return arm to side.			
3. Move arm across chest.			
4. Return arm to side.			
5. Move arm straight up.			

DATE SATISFACTORY DEMONSTRATION

INSTRUCTOR INITIALS

TOTAL HOURS FOR THIS CANDIDATE TO COMPLETE PROCEDURE

LOCATION

COMMENTS

(continued next page)

	DATE S/U	DATE S/U	DATE S/U
6. Return arm to side.			
7. Bring arm away from body at side to shoulder level			
8. Return arm to side.			
9. With arm straight out at the side, bend at elbow and rotate shoulder.			
10. Return arm to side.			
11. Bend at elbow and bring hand to chin.			
12. Return arm to side.			
C. Wrists, fingers and forearms:			
1. Bend hand backward at the wrist.			
2. Bend hand forward at the wrist.			
3. Clench fingers and thumb tightly as if making a fist.			
4. Extend fingers and thumb.			
5. Move fingers and thumb together and then apart.			
6. Flex and extend joints in thumb and fingers.			
7. Move each finger and thumb in a circular motion.			
8. Extend arm along side of body with palm facing upward.			
9. Rotate forearm with palm facing upward then downward.			
D. Legs, hips and knees:			
1. Stretch leg out from the body. Return leg to other leg crossing over other leg only at ankle.			
2. Bend and straighten knee.			
E. Ankles and toes:			
1. With leg straight on bed, push foot and toes toward front of leg.			

(continued next page)

	DATE S/U	DATE S/U	DATE S/U
2. Push foot and toes out straight with toes straight. Point towards foot of bed.			
3. With leg straight, turn foot and ankle from side to side.			
4. Curl toes downward and upward.			
9. Repeat each exercise as indicated on care plan.			
10. Note resident's response to exercise.			
11. Raise side rail. Lower bed.			
12. Place call light within resident's reach.			
13. Leave resident comfortable and safe.			
14. Tidy area.			
15. Wash your hands.			
16. Record or report resident's tolerance to procedure.			

Procedure 14

Brushing the Resident's Teeth

Name _____

Social Security Number _____

Certification Number _____

	DATE S/U	DATE S/U	DATE S/U
1. Wash your hands.			
2. Explain to resident who you are and what you are going to do.			
3. Gather supplies needed: toothbrush, toothpaste, water, mouthwash, emesis basin, towel, and disposable gloves.			
4. Place equipment on over-bed table.			
5. Give privacy.			
6. Raise bed to comfortable working height.			
7. Elevate head of bed.			
8. Lower side rail.			
9. Put on gloves.			
10. Place towel across resident's chest.			
11. Help resident in self-care, if possible.			
12. Moisten toothbrush. Apply toothpaste.			
13. Brush resident's teeth using circular motion to all surfaces. Brush gums, tongue, sides, and roof of mouth.			
14. Let resident rinse mouth with water or mouthwash.			
15. Hold emesis basin while resident spits.			
16. Wipe mouth with towel.			
17. Check mouth for sores, redness, or irritation.			
18. Raise side rail.			

DATE SATISFACTORY DEMONSTRATION

INSTRUCTOR INITIALS

TOTAL HOURS FOR THIS CANDIDATE TO COMPLETE PROCEDURE

LOCATION

COMMENTS

(continued next page)

	DATE S/U	DATE S/U	DATE S/U
19. Lower bed.			
20. Leave resident comfortable.			
21. Place call light within resident's reach.			
22. Clean and replace equipment.			
23. Wash your hands.			
24. Report or record the condition of mouth.			

Procedure **15**

Giving a Bed Bath

Name _____

Social Security Number _____

Certification Number _____

	DATE S/U	DATE S/U	DATE S/U	
1. Wash your hands.				**DATE SATISFACTORY DEMONSTRATION**
2. Explain to resident who you are and what you are going to do.				
3. Gather supplies needed: basin, soap, washcloth, two towels, clean gown, bath blanket, lotion, comb or brush, and gloves.				
4. Place supplies on clean area near bed.				**INSTRUCTOR INITIALS**
5. Check room temperature of room. Make sure resident is not cold.				
6. Give privacy.				
7. Offer bedpan or urinal to resident.				
8. Raise bed to comfortable working height.				
9. Lower side rail.				**TOTAL HOURS FOR THIS CANDIDATE TO COMPLETE PROCEDURE**
10. Remove bedspread and blanket. Fold them and place on chair.				
11. Place bath blanket over top sheet. Remove sheet without exposing resident. Place soiled sheet in hamper or on chair in room.				
12. Remove resident's gown.				
13. Raise side rail.				
14. Fill basin with warm water.				**LOCATION**
15. Return to bedside. Lower side rail.				
16. Place towel under chin.				**COMMENTS**
17. Offer washcloth to resident to wash own face, if possible.				

(continued next page)

	DATE S/U	DATE S/U	DATE S/U
18. Make a mitten by folding washcloth around your hand.			
19. Wash resident's eyelids from inner side of eye to outer side of eye.			
20. Rinse cloth.			
21. Wash face, neck, and ears.			
22. Dry washed areas.			
23. Place towel under resident's arm farthest from you.			
24. Hold resident's arm up. Wash the whole arm from wrist to shoulder.			
25. Rinse and dry arm.			
26. Wash, rinse, and dry axilla (armpit).			
27. Repeat for other arm.			
28. If possible, place resident's hands in water. Wash, rinse, and dry hands, fingers, and nails.			
29. Place towel across chest. Pull bath blanket down to abdomen.			
30. Move towel to expose chest.			
31. Wash, rinse, and dry chest.			
32. Cover chest with towel.			
33. Expose abdomen.			
34. Wash, rinse, and dry abdomen.			
35. Return bath blanket to resident's shoulders.			
36. Remove towel from under blanket.			
37. Uncover leg farthest from you. Place towel under leg.			
38. Wash, rinse, and dry leg.			
39. Repeat for other leg.			
40. If possible, place feet in basin one at a time.			
41. Wash, rinse, and dry feet.			

(continued next page)

	DATE S/U	DATE S/U	DATE S/U
42. Cover legs with bath blanket.			
43. Raise side rail.			
44. Empty basin and refill with clean water.			
45. Lower side rail.			
46. Ask resident to turn back toward you. Help him, if necessary.			
47. Wash, rinse, and dry back.			
48. Put lotion on back, massaging body prominences of hips, tailbone, spine, and shoulders.			
49. Use gloves to wash genital area. Wash from front of genital area to rectal area.			
50. Help resident into clean gown.			
51. Comb hair. Help with other grooming requests.			
52. Replace bed linens, if indicated.			
53. Position resident comfortably. Put call light within resident's reach.			
54. Raise side rail. Lower bed.			
55. Clean and replace equipment.			
56. Dispose of soiled linens.			
57. Wash your hands.			
58. Report or record skin condition and resident's tolerance.			

Procedure 16

Giving a Partial Bath With Perineal Care

Name _____

Social Security Number _____

Certification Number _____

	DATE S/U	DATE S/U	DATE S/U
1. Wash your hands.			
2. Explain to resident who you are and what you are going to do.			
3. Gather supplies needed: basin, soap, washcloth, two towels, bath blanket, clean gown or clothing, comb or brush, and gloves.			
4. Place supplies on clean area near bed.			
5. Check room temperature. Make sure resident is not cold.			
6. Give privacy.			
7. Offer bedpan or urinal to resident.			
8. Raise bed to comfortable working height.			
9. Lower side rail.			
10. Remove bedspread and blanket. Fold them and place on chair or fold at foot of bed.			
11. Place bath blanket over top sheet. Remove sheet without exposing resident. Place soiled sheet in hamper or on chair. Fold clean sheet to foot of bed.			
12. Raise side rail.			
13. Fill basin with warm water.			
14. Return to bedside. Lower side rail.			
15. Remove resident's gown.			
16. Place towel under chin.			
17. Offer washcloth to resident to wash own face, if possible.			

DATE SATISFACTORY DEMONSTRATION

INSTRUCTOR INITIALS

TOTAL HOURS FOR THIS CANDIDATE TO COMPLETE PROCEDURE

LOCATION

COMMENTS

(continued next page)

	DATE S/U	DATE S/U	DATE S/U
18. Make a mitten by folding washcloth around your hand.			
19. Wash resident's eyelids from inner side to outer side of eye.			
20. Rinse cloth.			
21. Wash face, neck, and ears.			
22. Dry washed areas.			
23. Place towel under hand farthest from you.			
24. If possible place resident's hand in basin. Wash, rinse, and dry hand.			
25. Repeat for other hand.			
26. Wash, rinse, and dry axilla (armpit).			
27. Repeat for other armpit.			
28. Help resident to turn his back to you.			
29. Wash, rinse, and dry upper back.			
30. Wash, rinse, and dry buttocks.			
31. Put lotion on back, massaging bony prominences of hips, tailbone, spine, and shoulders.			
32. Put on gloves.			
33. Wash perineal area.			
○ Female			
• Lift leg closer to you. Place on pillow, if necessary			
• Wash genital area from front to back, separating labia.			
• Wash area around anus last.			
• Rinse and dry very well.			
○ Male			
• Help him to lie on his back.			
• Wash penis, pubic area, and scrotum.			

(continued next page)

	DATE S/U	DATE S/U	DATE S/U
• If he is not circumcised, gently draw foreskin back and clean head of penis. Replace foreskin.			
• Rinse and dry very well.			
• Position male on his side to clean anus and anal area.			
34. Cover resident.			
35. Dress resident appropriately.			
36. Help grooming requests.			
37. Position resident comfortably. Put call light within resident's reach.			
38. Raise side rail. Lower bed.			
39. Clean and replace equipment.			
40. Throw out soiled linens.			
41. Wash your hands.			
42. Report or record resident's skin condition and tolerance.			

Procedure 17

Applying Lotion to the Resident

Name _____

Social Security Number _____

Certification Number _____

	DATE S/U	DATE S/U	DATE S/U
1. Wash your hands.			
2. Explain to resident who you are and what you are going to do.			
3. Gather supplies: lotion and towel.			
4. Provide privacy.			
5. Raise bed to working height.			
6. Lower side rail.			
7. Help resident turn on side, facing away from you.			
8. Expose back.			
9. Place towel along side of back.			
10. Pour small amount of lotion into hand, warm lotion with hand.			
11. Apply lotion to back. Pay special attention to bony prominences along spine, shoulders, hips, and tailbone.			
12. Continue to massage with smooth strokes until lotion is rubbed into skin.			
13. Wipe off extra lotion.			
14. Smooth and straighten bottom linens.			
15. Cover resident, and position him comfortably.			
16. If indicated, apply lotion to other pressure areas of skin, such as elbows and feet.			
17. Leave resident comfortable and safe.			
18. Place call light within resident's reach.			

DATE SATISFACTORY DEMONSTRATION

INSTRUCTOR INITIALS

TOTAL HOURS FOR THIS CANDIDATE TO COMPLETE PROCEDURE

LOCATION

COMMENTS

(continued next page)

	DATE S/U	DATE S/U	DATE S/U
19. Raise side rail.			
20. Lower bed.			
21. Tidy area. Throw away linens.			
22. Wash your hands.			
23. Record or report redness or skin irritation.			

Procedure 18

Applying Support Hosiery

Name _____

Social Security Number _____

Certification Number _____

	DATE S/U	DATE S/U	DATE S/U
1. Wash your hands.			
2. Explain to resident who you are and what you are going to do.			
3. Gather stockings of proper size.			
4. Give privacy.			
5. Help resident lie down.			
6. Expose one leg at a time.			
7. Grasp stocking with both hands at the top opening and roll or gather toward toe end.			
8. Adjust stocking over toes, foot, and heel.			
9. Apply stocking to leg by rolling or pulling upward over the leg.			
10. Make sure stocking is on evenly. Be sure there are no wrinkles.			
11. Expose other leg.			
12. Grasp stocking with both hands at the top opening and roll or gather toward toe end.			
13. Adjust stocking over toes, foot, and heel.			
14. Apply stocking to leg by rolling or pulling upward over the leg.			
15. Make sure stocking is on evenly. Be sure there are no wrinkles.			
16. Leave resident comfortable and safe.			
17. Place call light within resident's reach.			

DATE SATISFACTORY DEMONSTRATION

INSTRUCTOR INITIALS

TOTAL HOURS FOR THIS CANDIDATE TO COMPLETE PROCEDURE

LOCATION

COMMENTS

(continued next page)

	DATE S/U	DATE S/U	DATE S/U
18. Wash your hands.			
19. Report or record procedure.			

Procedure 19

Making the Occupied Bed

Name _____

Social Security Number _____

Certification Number _____

	DATE S/U	DATE S/U	DATE S/U	
1. Wash your hands.				**DATE SATISFACTORY DEMONSTRATION**
2. Explain to resident who you are and what you are going to do.				
3. Gather supplies needed: two large sheets, linen draw sheet, plastic or rubber draw sheet, bath blanket, pillow case, laundry bag or hamper, clean bedspread, and blanket, if needed.				
4. Hold linens away from your uniform.				**INSTRUCTOR INITIALS**
5. Place supplies on clean area near bed in order of use. From top to bottom: pillow case, spread, sheet, linen draw sheet, plastic or rubber draw sheet, and sheets.				
6. Provide privacy for resident.				
7. Raise bed to comfortable working height. Lock wheels of bed.				
8. Lower side rail on working side. Make sure other side rail is secure.				**TOTAL HOURS FOR THIS CANDIDATE TO COMPLETE PROCEDURE**
9. Remove bedspread and blanket. Fold and place on chair.				
10. Place bath blanket over top sheet. Remove sheet without exposing resident. Place soiled sheet in hamper or on chair in room. Or, if not using bath blanket, leave top sheet covering resident.				
11. Help resident to turn on side away from you.				**LOCATION**
12. Loosen bottom linens.				
13. Roll soiled draw sheet and rubber sheet and tuck along resident's back.				**COMMENTS**
14. Roll soiled bottom sheet and tuck along resident's back under the draw sheet and rubber sheet.				

(continued next page)

	DATE S/U	DATE S/U	DATE S/U
15. Place clean sheet on bed with center fold at center of bed.			
16. Unfold one half of sheet.			
17. Place bottom hem of sheet even with edge of mattress. Or, fit corner of fitted sheet.			
18. Tuck top of sheet under half of head end of mattress.			
19. Miter corner of top sheet. Or, fit corner of fitted sheet.			
20. Tuck sheet under side of entire mattress, working from head to foot of bed.			
21. Roll remaining half of sheet and tuck under soiled sheet.			
22. Place rubber draw sheet in the middle of bed. Tuck in at side of bed.			
23. Place clean linen draw sheet over rubber draw sheet. Tuck in at side of bed.			
24. Roll remaining halves of draw sheets and tuck along resident's back under the soiled sheets.			
25. Help resident roll over linen pile to side facing you.			
26. Raise side rail.			
27. Go to other side of bed.			
28. Lower side rail.			
29. Loosen and remove soiled linens from under mattress.			
30. Place soiled linens on chair or in hamper. *Do not put linens on floor.*			
31. Pull clean bottom sheet over mattress.			
32. Tuck the bottom sheet tight under head of mattress.			
33. Miter corner of sheet at head of bed. Or, fit corner of fitted sheet.			
34. Pull bottom sheet tight, and tuck under side of mattress, working from head to foot of bed.			

(continued next page)

	DATE S/U	DATE S/U	DATE S/U
35. Pull rubber sheet tight, and tuck over bottom sheet at side of mattress.			
36. Pull draw sheet tight, and tuck over rubber sheet at side of mattress.			
37. Help the resident to roll on back. Place bath blanket or bed sheet on resident.			
38. Place clean sheet over bath blanket or bed sheet, centering center fold of sheet.			
39. Pull bath blanket or soiled sheet from under clean sheet.			
40. Place blanket and bedspread over sheet.			
41. Fold top sheet over edge of blanket. Spread to make a cuff with sheet.			
42. Tuck top linens under foot of mattress, giving "toe room" for resident's feet.			
43. Miter the corner of top linens at foot of bed.			
44. Raise side rail.			
45. Go to other side of bed.			
46. Tuck top linens under mattress at foot of bed.			
47. Miter corner of top linens at foot of bed, giving "toe room" for resident's feet.			
48. Remove pillow and soiled pillowcase.			
49. Place clean pillowcase on pillow.			
50. Replace pillow under resident's head.			
51. Leave resident comfortable and safe.			
52. Place call light within resident's reach.			
53. Raise side rail.			
54. Lower bed.			
55. Tidy area. Put linens in hamper.			
56. Wash your hands.			
57. Record or report resident's tolerance to procedure.			

Procedure 20

Feeding the Resident

Name

Social Security Number

Certification Number

	DATE S/U	DATE S/U	DATE S/U	
1. Wash your hands.				**DATE SATISFACTORY DEMONSTRATION**
2. Explain to resident who you are and what you are going to do.				
3. Offer resident help with toileting.				
4. Position resident in comfortable sitting position in bed or chair.				
5. Position over-bed table over resident's lap.				
6. Check meal tray for silverware, spilled foods.				**INSTRUCTOR INITIALS**
7. Gather adaptive equipment, if necessary: napkin or towel, long-handled spoon, plate guard, or non-spill cup, etc.				
8. Make sure it is the correct menu for the resident.				
9. Place tray on table. Remove food covers.				**TOTAL HOURS FOR THIS CANDIDATE TO COMPLETE PROCEDURE**
10. Sit near resident.				
11. Explain what is on tray.				
12. Ask resident what foods he would like to eat first.				
13. Encourage resident to feed himself, if able, by using finger foods or adaptive equipment.				
14. Use hand-on-hand technique to help resident to feed himself.				**LOCATION**
15. Fill fork or spoon only half full or less, according to resident's ability to swallow.				**COMMENTS**
16. Use straw for liquids.				
17. Encourage resident. Talk pleasantly. Do not rush resident.				

(continued next page)

	DATE S/U	DATE S/U	DATE S/U
18. Wipe resident's mouth.			
19. Offer liquids between amounts of solid food.			
20. Remove tray when resident is finished.			
21. Wash resident's hands, if necessary.			
22. Replace side rail if it is lowered.			
23. Leave resident comfortable.			
24. Place call light within resident's reach.			
25. Note amount of food and fluids taken, according to facility procedure.			
26. Wash your hands.			
27. Record or report amounts of food and fluid taken in. Record percentage or fractions on intake and output sheet. Note resident's eating, chewing, and self-help ability.			

Procedure 21 ————————————

Recording Intake and Output

Name _____

Social Security Number _____

Certification Number _____

	DATE S/U	DATE S/U	DATE S/U
1. Wash your hands.			
2. Explain to resident who you are and what you are going to do.			
3. Check to identify equivalents used in your facility (e.g. coffee cup (5 oz) = 150 cc, glass (8 oz) = 240 cc)			
4. Identify foods taken by resident that are considered liquid.			
5. Estimate the amount of liquid food taken.			
6. Record on I&O sheet in cubic centi-meters the amount of liquid foods taken by resident.			
7. Record amounts under intake column.			
8. Measure output of resident by pouring contents of urinal, bedpan, or emesis basin into graduate (measuring pitcher).			
9. Record the output in cubic centimeters in the appropriate column.			
10. Leave resident comfortable and safe with call light within resident's reach.			
11. Wash your hands.			
12. Return meal tray to appropriate area.			
13. Report or record, as indicated by facility policy.			

DATE SATISFACTORY DEMONSTRATION

INSTRUCTOR INITIALS

TOTAL HOURS FOR THIS CANDIDATE TO COMPLETE PROCEDURE

LOCATION

COMMENTS

Procedure 22

Giving a Bedpan

Name _____

Social Security Number _____

Certification Number _____

	DATE S/U	DATE S/U	DATE S/U
1. Wash your hands.			
2. Explain to resident who you are and what you are going to do.			
3. Gather supplies: bedpan, bedpan cover, and tissue.			
4. Give privacy.			
5. Raise bed to working height. Lower head of bed.			
6. Lower side rail on working side.			
7. Fold upper linen down to expose resident's buttocks.			
8. Place your hands on resident's shoulder and hip. Log roll (turn with resident's body in a straight line) resident to side away from you. Resident may help to turn by grasping side rail away from you. *Or,* ask resident to bend legs and raise buttocks.			
9. Place bedpan so wider end of pan is aligned with resident's buttocks.			
10. Hold pan in place while turning resident onto back if resident has been turned to side.			
11. Cover resident.			
12. Raise side rail.			
13. Lower bed. Raise headrest unless resident must remain flat.			
14. Place call light and tissue within reach of resident.			
15. Leave room. Assure the resident's privacy.			

DATE SATISFACTORY DEMONSTRATION

INSTRUCTOR INITIALS

TOTAL HOURS FOR THIS CANDIDATE TO COMPLETE PROCEDURE

LOCATION

COMMENTS

(continued next page)

	DATE S/U	DATE S/U	DATE S/U
16. Return when called by resident.			
17. Gather supplies, if necessary, to clean perineal area of resident: gloves, basin of warm water, washcloth, and towel.			
18. Lower head of bed. Raise bed to working level, lower side rail.			
19. Fold covers back to expose resident's buttocks.			
20. Turn resident on side away from you, place one hand on shoulder, and one hand on hip. *Or,* ask resident to bend legs and lift buttocks.			
21. Hold bedpan while resident is turning or lifting.			
22. Remove, cover, and place bedpan near foot of bed or on chair.			
23. Put on gloves to wipe perineal area.			
24. Clean perineal area with toilet tissue, if resident is unable.			
25. Wash perineal area with warm, wet washcloth.			
26. Rinse and dry perineal area very well.			
27. Check skin for redness or irritation.			
28. Turn resident to back.			
29. Cover resident.			
30. Position resident comfortably.			
31. Raise side rail. Lower bed.			
32. Empty contents of bedpan into toilet or graduate (measuring pitcher).			
33. If resident is on I&O, measure urine.			
34. Clean bedpan. Cover it and replace to proper area.			
35. Wash your hands.			
36. Help resident wash his hands.			
37. Leave resident comfortable and safe.			

(continued next page)

	DATE S/U	DATE S/U	DATE S/U
38. Place call light within resident's reach.			
39. Record or report output. Note color, amount, or anything unusual. Record condition of resident's skin.			

Procedure 23

Giving Catheter Care

Name _____

Social Security Number _____

Certification Number _____

	DATE S/U	DATE S/U	DATE S/U
1. Wash your hands.			
2. Explain to resident who you are and what you are going to do.			
3. Gather supplies: basin of warm water, washcloth, towel, gloves, tape or rubber band, and pin			
4. Give privacy.			
5. Raise bed to working height.			
6. Lower side rail on working side.			
7. Fold top linen down to expose catheter.			
8. Observe tubing for urine flow, pressure, secure connections, and kinks.			
9. Put on gloves.			
10. Wash urethra area around catheter entrance.			
11. Wash genital area from front area to back. Rinse often.			
12. Dry area very well.			
13. Secure or attach catheter, according to care plan.			
14. Place drainage tubing over resident's leg.			
15. Place tape or rubber band around tubing and pin tape or rubber band to sheet at edge of mattress to make sure that extra tubing stays on bed.			
16. Cover resident.			
17. Raise side rail. Lower bed.			

DATE SATISFACTORY DEMONSTRATION

INSTRUCTOR INITIALS

TOTAL HOURS FOR THIS CANDIDATE TO COMPLETE PROCEDURE

LOCATION

COMMENTS

(continued next page)

	DATE S/U	DATE S/U	DATE S/U
18. Empty drainage bag. Open clamp on bag. Let urine drain into a graduate. This is usually done at end of shift.			
19. Record amount of urine.			
20. Make sure drainage bag is lower than bladder and attached securely to bed frame.			
21. Check tubing to make sure urine is flowing.			
22. Leave resident comfortable and safe.			
23. Place call light within resident's reach.			
24. Wash your hands.			
25. Record or report output. Note color, amount, and anything unusual.			

Procedure 24

Taking the Oral Temperature

Name _____

Social Security Number _____

Certification Number _____

	DATE S/U	DATE S/U	DATE S/U
1. Wash your hands.			
2. Explain to resident who you are and what you are going to do.			
3. Gather supplies: oral thermometer, watch with a second hand, pencil and paper, tissue, and gloves.			
4. Rinse thermometer with cold water and wipe with tissue from stem to mercury bulb end, if thermometer has been in disinfectant.			
5. Read thermometer. Shake down to 96°F.			
6. Ask resident if he has had hot or cold liquids or smoked a cigarette. If so, wait 10 minutes.			
7. Place bulb of thermometer under resident's tongue.			
8. Ask resident to close lips and breathe through nose.			
9. Note time of insertion and remove in 5 minutes or time interval on facility policy.			
10. Wipe thermometer from stem to bulb with tissue.			
11. Read thermometer to nearest two tenths of a degree.			
12. Record temperature on paper.			
13. Clean thermometer, if indicated, or replace in container.			
14. Leave resident comfortable and safe.			
15. Place call light within resident's reach.			
16. Wash your hands.			

DATE
SATISFACTORY
DEMONSTRATION

INSTRUCTOR
INITIALS

TOTAL HOURS FOR
THIS CANDIDATE
TO COMPLETE
PROCEDURE

LOCATION

COMMENTS

(continued next page)

	DATE S/U	DATE S/U	DATE S/U
17. Record on sheet according to facility policy.			
18. Report any unusual temperature to nurse.			

Procedure 25

Taking the Pulse and Respirations

Name _____

Social Security Number _____

Certification Number _____

	DATE S/U	DATE S/U	DATE S/U
1. Wash your hands.			
2. Explain to the resident who you are and what you want to do. Tell the resident you are taking the pulse. Do not tell resident that you are going to count respirations.			
3. Gather supplies: watch with a second hand, and pencil and paper.			
4. Position resident's arm on flat surface. Ask resident to relax arm.			
5. Place tips of 2 or 3 of your fingers on the palm and thumb side of resident's wrist.			
6. Locate pulse with your fingers.			
7. Do not use thumb to feel pulse.			
8. Press lightly with fingers to feel pulse.			
9. Look at the position of second hand on watch.			
10. Count and remember the pulse beats for 30 seconds. Note volume and rhythm. Count for 1 minute, if pulse is irregular.			
11. Continue to hold the resident's wrist as if you are still taking the pulse count.			
12. Observe the rising and falling of the resident's chest.			
13. Count one rise and one fall of chest as one respiration.			
14. Count for 30 seconds. Note regularity. Count for 1 minute if respirations are irregular.			
15. Remove your hand from resident's wrist.			

DATE SATISFACTORY DEMONSTRATION

INSTRUCTOR INITIALS

TOTAL HOURS FOR THIS CANDIDATE TO COMPLETE PROCEDURE

LOCATION

COMMENTS

(continued next page)

	DATE S/U	DATE S/U	DATE S/U
16. Multiply by two the number of pulse beats, if counted for 30 seconds.			
17. Record on paper the 1-minute pulse.			
18. Multiply by two the number of respirations, if counted for 30 seconds.			
19. Record on paper the 1-minute respirations.			
20. Leave resident comfortable and safe.			
21. Place call light within resident's reach.			
22. Wash your hands.			
23. Record on sheet according to facility policy.			
24. Report any unusual findings to nurse.			

Procedure **26**

Taking the Blood Pressure

Name _____

Social Security Number _____

Certification Number _____

	DATE S/U	DATE S/U	DATE S/U
1. Wash your hands.			
2. Explain to resident who you are and what you want to do. Tell the resident this is not a painful procedure, but he or she may feel some tingling or numbness in arm.			
3. Gather supplies: sphygmomanometer with proper cuff size, stethoscope, pencil and paper, and alcohol wipes.			
4. Check earpieces of stethoscope. Clean with alcohol wipes.			
5. Help resident to comfortable position in bed or chair.			
6. Remove or loosen clothing from arm.			
7. Place arm in comfortable position on flat surface.			
8. Locate the brachial artery.			
9. Make sure cuff is decompressed.			
10. Wrap cuff snugly and smoothly around upper arm. Place it about one inch above bend of elbow. The inflatable portion of the cuff must be over brachial artery.			
11. Make sure tubing from cuff is centered.			
12. Place earpieces of stethoscope in your ears.			
13. Relocate the brachial artery.			
14. Place diaphragm of stethoscope over brachial artery.			
15. Hold stethoscope in place tightly against skin.			

DATE SATISFACTORY DEMONSTRATION

INSTRUCTOR INITIALS

TOTAL HOURS FOR THIS CANDIDATE TO COMPLETE PROCEDURE

LOCATION

COMMENTS

(continued next page)

	DATE S/U	DATE S/U	DATE S/U
16. Tighten clockwise the thumb screw of valve on rubber bulb with other hand.			
17. Squeeze rubber bulb to inflate the cuff and to raise dial of mercury to approximately 160-170 mm or as indicated on care plan.			
18. Open thumb screw of valve just enough to hear air escape. Allow dial or mercury to slowly go down, dropping about 2mm per beat.			
19. Watch gauge carefully and listen for first clear sound of regular beats.			
20. Read and remember column or dial number of the systolic reading.			
21. Let air continue escaping slowly.			
22. Listen carefully for the last sound.			
23. Read and remember column or dial at this point for the diastolic reading.			
24. Loosen thumb screw quickly and let all the air out of inflatable cuff.			
25. Remove cuff from resident's arm.			
26. Remove stethoscope from ears.			
27. Record readings in fraction format on paper.			
28. Leave resident comfortable and safe.			
29. Place call light within resident's reach.			
30. Clean earpieces of stethoscope with alcohol wipes.			
31. Wash your hands.			
32. Replace equipment.			
33. Record on sheet according to facility policy.			
34. Report any unusual findings to nurse.			

Appendix **D** _____

Practice Answer Sheet

1. (A) (B) (C) (D)
2. (A) (B) (C) (D)
3. (A) (B) (C) (D)
4. (A) (B) (C) (D)
5. (A) (B) (C) (D)
6. (A) (B) (C) (D)
7. (A) (B) (C) (D)
8. (A) (B) (C) (D)
9. (A) (B) (C) (D)
10. (A) (B) (C) (D)
11. (A) (B) (C) (D)
12. (A) (B) (C) (D)
13. (A) (B) (C) (D)
14. (A) (B) (C) (D)
15. (A) (B) (C) (D)
16. (A) (B) (C) (D)
17. (A) (B) (C) (D)
18. (A) (B) (C) (D)
19. (A) (B) (C) (D)
20. (A) (B) (C) (D)
21. (A) (B) (C) (D)
22. (A) (B) (C) (D)
23. (A) (B) (C) (D)
24. (A) (B) (C) (D)
25. (A) (B) (C) (D)
26. (A) (B) (C) (D)
27. (A) (B) (C) (D)
28. (A) (B) (C) (D)
29. (A) (B) (C) (D)
30. (A) (B) (C) (D)
31. (A) (B) (C) (D)
32. (A) (B) (C) (D)
33. (A) (B) (C) (D)
34. (A) (B) (C) (D)
35. (A) (B) (C) (D)
36. (A) (B) (C) (D)
37. (A) (B) (C) (D)
38. (A) (B) (C) (D)
39. (A) (B) (C) (D)
40. (A) (B) (C) (D)

41. (A) (B) (C) (D)
42. (A) (B) (C) (D)
43. (A) (B) (C) (D)
44. (A) (B) (C) (D)
45. (A) (B) (C) (D)
46. (A) (B) (C) (D)
47. (A) (B) (C) (D)
48. (A) (B) (C) (D) (E)
49. (A) (B) (C) (D)
50. (A) (B) (C) (D)
51. (A) (B) (C) (D)
52. (A) (B) (C) (D)
53. (A) (B) (C) (D)
54. (A) (B) (C) (D)
55. (A) (B) (C) (D)
56. (A) (B) (C) (D)
57. (A) (B) (C) (D)
58. (A) (B) (C) (D)
59. (A) (B) (C) (D)
60. (A) (B) (C) (D)
61. (A) (B) (C) (D)
62. (A) (B) (C) (D)
63. (A) (B) (C) (D)
64. (A) (B) (C) (D)
65. (A) (B) (C) (D)
66. (A) (B) (C) (D)
67. (A) (B) (C) (D)
68. (A) (B) (C) (D)
69. (A) (B) (C) (D)
70. (A) (B) (C) (D)
71. (A) (B) (C) (D)
72. (A) (B) (C) (D)
73. (A) (B) (C) (D)
74. (A) (B) (C) (D)
75. (A) (B) (C) (D)

Appendix **D** _____

Practice Answer Sheet

1. (A) (B) (C) (D)
2. (A) (B) (C) (D)
3. (A) (B) (C) (D)
4. (A) (B) (C) (D)
5. (A) (B) (C) (D)
6. (A) (B) (C) (D)
7. (A) (B) (C) (D)
8. (A) (B) (C) (D)
9. (A) (B) (C) (D)
10. (A) (B) (C) (D)
11. (A) (B) (C) (D)
12. (A) (B) (C) (D)
13. (A) (B) (C) (D)
14. (A) (B) (C) (D)
15. (A) (B) (C) (D)
16. (A) (B) (C) (D)
17. (A) (B) (C) (D)
18. (A) (B) (C) (D)
19. (A) (B) (C) (D)
20. (A) (B) (C) (D)
21. (A) (B) (C) (D)
22. (A) (B) (C) (D)
23. (A) (B) (C) (D)
24. (A) (B) (C) (D)
25. (A) (B) (C) (D)
26. (A) (B) (C) (D)
27. (A) (B) (C) (D)
28. (A) (B) (C) (D)
29. (A) (B) (C) (D)
30. (A) (B) (C) (D)
31. (A) (B) (C) (D)
32. (A) (B) (C) (D)
33. (A) (B) (C) (D)
34. (A) (B) (C) (D)
35. (A) (B) (C) (D)
36. (A) (B) (C) (D)
37. (A) (B) (C) (D)
38. (A) (B) (C) (D)
39. (A) (B) (C) (D)
40. (A) (B) (C) (D)

41. (A) (B) (C) (D)
42. (A) (B) (C) (D)
43. (A) (B) (C) (D)
44. (A) (B) (C) (D)
45. (A) (B) (C) (D)
46. (A) (B) (C) (D)
47. (A) (B) (C) (D)
48. (A) (B) (C) (D) (E)
49. (A) (B) (C) (D)
50. (A) (B) (C) (D)
51. (A) (B) (C) (D)
52. (A) (B) (C) (D)
53. (A) (B) (C) (D)
54. (A) (B) (C) (D)
55. (A) (B) (C) (D)
56. (A) (B) (C) (D)
57. (A) (B) (C) (D)
58. (A) (B) (C) (D)
59. (A) (B) (C) (D)
60. (A) (B) (C) (D)
61. (A) (B) (C) (D)
62. (A) (B) (C) (D)
63. (A) (B) (C) (D)
64. (A) (B) (C) (D)
65. (A) (B) (C) (D)
66. (A) (B) (C) (D)
67. (A) (B) (C) (D)
68. (A) (B) (C) (D)
69. (A) (B) (C) (D)
70. (A) (B) (C) (D)
71. (A) (B) (C) (D)
72. (A) (B) (C) (D)
73. (A) (B) (C) (D)
74. (A) (B) (C) (D)
75. (A) (B) (C) (D)

Index